Eat.
Lift.
Thrive.

Sohee Lee

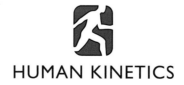

HUMAN KINETICS

Library of Congress Info

Names: Lee, Sohee, 1989- author.
Title: Eat. Lift. Thrive. / Sohee Lee.
Description: Champaign, IL : Human Kinetics, [2017] | Includes
  bibliographical references and index.
Identifiers: LCCN 2017017225 (print) | LCCN 2016050380 (ebook) | ISBN
  9781492545910 (ebook) | ISBN 9781492545903 (print)
Subjects: LCSH: Women--Health and hygiene. | Physical fitness for women.
Classification: LCC RA778 (print) | LCC RA778 .L464 2017 (ebook) | DDC
  613.7/045--dc23
LC record available at https://lccn.loc.gov/2017017225
ISBN: 978-1-4925-4590-3 (print)

This publication is written and published to provide accurate and authoritative information relevant to the subject matter presented. It is published and sold with the understanding that the author and publisher are not engaged in rendering legal, medical, or other professional services by reason of their authorship or publication of this work. If medical or other expert assistance is required, the services of a competent professional person should be sought.

The web addresses cited in this text were current as of February 2017, unless otherwise noted.

Acquisitions Editor: Michelle Maloney; **Senior Developmental Editor:** Cynthia McEntire; **Managing Editor:** Caitlin Husted; **Copyeditor:** Bob Replinger; **Indexer:** Andrea Hepner; **Permissions Manager:** Martha Gullo; **Senior Graphic Designer:** Joe Buck; **Cover Designer:** Keri Evans; **Photograph (cover):** © Human Kinetics; **Photographs (interior):** © Human Kinetics; **Visual Production Assistant:** Joyce Brumfield; **Photo Production Manager:** Jason Allen; **Models:** Sohee Lee, Hyla Conrad, Karey Northington, Shelley Cook; **Senior Art Manager:** Kelly Hendren; **Illustrations:** © Human Kinetics; **Printer:** Versa Press

We thank Eric and Karey Northington for their assistance in providing the location for the photo shoot for this book.

Human Kinetics books are available at special discounts for bulk purchase. Special editions or book excerpts can also be created to specification. For details, contact the Special Sales Manager at Human Kinetics.

Printed in the United States of America

10 9 8 7 6 5 4 3 2 1

The paper in this book is certified under a sustainable forestry program.

Human Kinetics

Website: www.HumanKinetics.com

United States: Human Kinetics
P.O. Box 5076
Champaign, IL 61825-5076
800-747-4457
e-mail: info@hkusa.com

Canada: Human Kinetics
475 Devonshire Road Unit 100
Windsor, ON N8Y 2L5
800-465-7301 (in Canada only)
e-mail: info@hkcanada.com

Europe: Human Kinetics
107 Bradford Road
Stanningley
Leeds LS28 6AT, United Kingdom
+44 (0) 113 255 5665
e-mail: hk@hkeurope.com

For information about Human Kinetics' coverage in other areas of the world, please visit our website: www.HumanKinetics.com

E7002

I dedicate this book to my Umma and Abba for fostering my love for learning and to my mentors, Bret Contreras and Layne Norton, for believing in my potential, encouraging me to pursue my passion, and gently nudging me into the world of science.

CONTENTS

FOREWORD

When it comes to the fitness industry, I don't envy women. Not because I think men are superior or that women are somehow inferior—quite the contrary. I don't envy women because they come into this industry facing more assumptions, expectations, pressure, and, quite frankly, nonsense compared to men. Ladies, at what age were you first told that you should be skinny? When was the first time you felt compelled to go on a diet? When was the first time you were made to feel guilty for having a "bad" food? For many of you, this would have occurred before the age of 10. Most males don't think about such things before high school or even later.

As a coach, I receive e-mails every week from women broken by the fitness industry. They don't feel good enough, they aren't fit enough, they aren't skinny enough, they don't eat clean enough. Why can't they look like their favorite fitness models, no matter how hard they try? Why does it feel like the harder they work, the further away from their goals they get?

Instead of helping these women build more confidence and improve health, and directing them to the correct things, the fitness industry attempts to exploit insecurities for a profit. Confidence is bad for business, because being happy with yourself doesn't sell. After all, if you feel good about yourself, why do you need what Joe Schmoe fitness guru is trying to sell you? Week after week, I'm inundated with e-mails from women who have tried every fad diet, supplement, six-week challenge, weird piece of fitness equipment, and new "it" workout in an effort to find the magic piece of the puzzle. The result of this journey is an emotional roller coaster that leaves them bitter and hopeless, with their fitness goals sliding further away from them.

I've been blessed to see women make their way back from rock bottom. To not only improve their physiques, but to reach a point where they were so confident going through the journey of fitness that they didn't care about other people's opinions or judgments. Where they could crush weights during the day, have plenty of energy, and eat a piece of chocolate at night without feeling guilty or gorging on the whole bag.

The balance of mental fitness with physical fitness is often overlooked. I know plenty of women with ripped physiques who are beasts in the gym. Would I consider the majority of them healthy? Honestly, after working with many of them, I wouldn't. Even if you have a six-pack and can squat 250 pounds, are you really healthy if you call yourself fat, can't be happy in a relationship, constantly compare yourself to others, receive your validation only through likes on Instagram, and struggle daily with an eating disorder? No, I certainly wouldn't consider you healthy. There are women who achieve the balance of overall mental and physical fitness, but it's not easy. Most women don't even know where to start.

Enter Sohee Lee. I was fortunate to meet Sohee early in her fitness journey. She was a young writer who wanted to interview me for her blog, and I was impressed with her approach to fitness and health. Her struggles with self-image and food issues pushed her to learn more in an effort to help others. At the time we met, I was drowning in client e-mails, and my business was growing so rapidly that I needed help. Sohee reached out to me, never asking for payment in return for becoming my assistant (of course, I paid her), and she made a huge difference to me. I knew that I wouldn't be able to keep her as my assistant for long. She was too smart, too talented, and too driven to settle for being an assistant. When she was ready to step out on her own, I couldn't have been more proud. And as my cohost on the podcast *Physique Science Radio*, she offers perspectives and insights, often from the mental health perspective, which I would never consider.

Sohee has a bachelor's degree in human biology, has won her bikini pro card, has written books, and has coached many clients successfully. But these accolades are not what make her great. What makes Sohee great is her commitment to giving back to others. In fact, she is currently pursuing a master's degree in psychology. She doesn't need this degree; she was already well on the path to a thriving career, I assure you. She is doing it because she feels driven to do it. She's curious. She has questions that will not be answered unless she takes the initiative to answer them. This is what makes the core of great evidence-based practitioners: the will to put themselves to the fire, learn more, and be humbled in the process. And believe me, graduate school is an incredibly humbling process.

It is for this reason alone—her compulsion to give back—that I would ask you to read this book. But if you need more reasons, then I will be happy to tell you that within these pages are the answers to the questions you have, and to those you didn't even know you had. She's not going to lie to you. She's not going to sell you false hope. If you are looking for a six-week challenge to get ripped, you've come to the wrong place. If you've come here to find out what the 10 magic foods for getting a six-pack are, go ahead and put this book down; it's not for you. But if you've come to learn how to achieve real and sustainable results, keep reading. Sohee will provide you with the blueprint to turn fitness into a sustainable lifestyle. You must enter with an open mind; much of this book will be different than what you are used to hearing. Even more important, she does not address just physiological aspects of the fitness journey, but also psychological aspects, which are often more important.

Welcome to the journey. Welcome to the movement. Welcome to *Eat. Lift. Thrive.*

Dr. Layne Norton
Bodybuilding and physique coach
Founder of Carbon & BioLayne LLC
Professional powerlifter
IFPA all-natural bodybuilder

PREFACE

"I can't figure out this nutrition thing!"

"I know what to do, but I just can't seem to apply the right behaviors consistently."

"I can get lean, but I can't stay lean."

"I'm tired of yo-yo dieting; I want to keep this body fat off for life."

These are just a few of the responses I received when I asked my readers to name their biggest struggle with fitness. You'll notice that none of the remarks had anything to do with exercise or training per se; instead, they were about nutrition and behavior change as a whole.

This focus comes as no surprise to me.

We don't have a weight-loss problem; in fact, we are remarkably good at shedding weight and doing so quickly. The issue is more with keeping that weight off over the long haul. In fact, more than 95 percent of people who lose weight gain it back eventually (McGuire et al. 1999). How disheartening is that?

On any given day, we are presented with countless opportunities to eat food, and we have an infinite number of options. What to eat? How much? When? And then what?

What makes nutrition so complex is that, despite what others may tell you, it's far more than just fuel. Depending on your culture, eating may be a form of social glue, a love language of sorts. It's also deeply connected to memories. When I think of sweetened condensed milk, for example, I'm immediately taken back to my childhood, standing in my in-line skates with the fridge door wide open as I poured the can of sweet sugary goodness straight into my mouth. Yeesh! But what a wonderful time of my life that was. So, yes, comfort food is a real thing. Our emotions are acutely intertwined with food.

This book is for those of you who feel overwhelmed by the plethora of information surrounding nutrition and exercise; for those of you who know what to do in theory but have trouble applying fat-loss principles consistently.

You probably know what protein, carbohydrate, and fat are (if not, don't worry), but you're not sure what to do with that information. Maybe you don't believe that weighing every morsel of food you consume and plugging it into a nutrition app is the only way to be fit (hint: It's not). Maybe you've heard of the idea of intuitive eating but don't trust yourself enough to give it a worthwhile shot.

Before I discovered lifting weights, I was instructed to perform sit-ups for one hour straight every morning on an empty stomach followed immediately by power walking for another hour to obtain a svelte physique. Another acquaintance looked me straight in the eyes and said that the slower I walked, the more body fat I would burn. Therefore, I should move in slow motion at all times. You can't make this up! You've likely received similar well-intentioned, yet ludicrous, recommendations from friends, family, and colleagues about how to get abs and slim your thighs.

All of this may seem confusing, and understandably so. Contrary to popular belief, you don't have to become a slave to the treadmill, and you don't have to dread your workouts to feel confident in your own skin. I'll teach you about the seemingly magical power of resistance training, and I'll show you how chasing strength in the gym can transform your life in more ways than one. It's not about logging more hours; it's about training smarter. You can build muscle and shed body fat with as little as three to four hours of exercise per week if you follow my methods.

Here's the deal: Moderation isn't glamorous. We're almost disappointed when we find out that someone we know lost a good deal of body fat and improved her health simply by practicing consistent moderation. What? That's it? We look for heroics; we love extreme measures.

But here's the other deal: Moderation is freakin' hard. In fact, the easier approach is to grab one extreme and then catapult to another, lurching back and forth in a race to reach the final destination as quickly as possible. Ironically, this method has us spinning our wheels and getting nowhere fast.

Wouldn't it be nice for nutrition to feel effortless?

Wouldn't it be incredible to be able to go on vacation, or even just out to a restaurant, and enjoy your meals without anxiety?

Wouldn't it be wonderful to stay lean year round, not cut your favorite foods from your diet, and enjoy your life while you're at it?

Does all this sound too good to be true? It's not.

I've come to learn that knowing the facts won't do you any good unless you can learn the practical tools that allow you to apply the right behaviors to your life consistently. For that to happen, you need to get your mindset right before the pieces of the puzzle can fall neatly into place.

This book will teach you to reframe the way you think about food and exercise.

IT ALL STARTS WITH UNDERSTANDING BEHAVIOR CHANGE

We glamorize heroics: We laud grandiose journeys of lifestyle transformation. These stories make headlines, and they pass from friend to friend like wildfire. Did you hear that Sally dropped 50 pounds (23 kg) in a span of two months eating nothing but cabbage? Did you know that Jerry lost six pants sizes in three weeks on the honey-and-lemon diet? You should try it, my dear!

So inspirational. If only we could be like them.

Of course, we might reason that because other people have seemingly willed their way to skinny by extreme methods, we can do the same.

But lasting behavior change is about more than simply making the decision to do something different. It's about more than wanting something badly enough or writing a plan down on paper.

All the facts in the world won't mean a thing if you don't have the tools to use them. Knowledge does not automatically translate into application.

Fat loss, and any worthwhile health behavior change for that matter, begins with the mind. Of course, not everyone here is on a quest to lose body fat per se. Maybe you care more about your overall health, and you want to be able to run after your grandkids in your later years without running out of breath. Perhaps you simply want to be able to walk up a flight of stairs without getting winded. Or you may just want to feel confident in your own skin again. All of that is more than fine.

Whatever it is you want to accomplish, it all starts with habits.

We'll be discussing habits a lot in this book. We all know what habits are: A routine or behavior that occurs regularly and seemingly automatically. The *American Journal of Psychology* defines it as a "fixed way of thinking, willing, or feeling acquired through previous repetition of a mental experience" (Andrew 1903).

A habit could be as minor as twirling a pen in your fingers when you're on the phone or as deleterious for your health as smoking. Some habits are good for you, whereas others can wreak havoc on your system. Habits comprise most of our actions throughout each day, allowing us to repeat patterns of behavior without conscious thought.

Habits lie at the crux of behavior change. If you understand how to use habits to work in your favor, your chances of achieving a long-term lifestyle change are far greater.

WHITE-KNUCKLING IS NOT THE ANSWER

I once mistakenly believed that if only I had an unlimited supply of self-control, I could achieve the body I wanted. I thought I'd consume a perfect diet full of high-quality meats and grains and vegetables and scoff at added sugars and grease. I assumed I'd happily pedal away on the stationary bike at the gym with a thousand-watt smile plastered on my face the whole time.

If I ever slipped up with my fitness, I reprimanded myself for not trying harder. I would then further tighten the reins and be even stricter with myself, only to shoot myself in the foot, again. Still, I figured that if I simply used enough brute force, I would finally get to where I wanted to be.

But it wasn't fun, and it certainly wasn't easy. I even came to a point where I wondered whether I simply didn't have it in me to be lean at all. I stared longingly at my thinner friends as they shimmied around in size-zero jeans and confidently rocked teeny-weeny bikinis. They obviously had more willpower than I did to be able to look that way all the time—or so I thought.

Lasting behavior change actually has less to do with self-control than we believe. White-knuckling your way to long-term lifestyle modification, in other words, is the harder and less successful way to go about things. You don't have to, and shouldn't, rely on mindless, exhaustive efforts to accomplish a fitness goal. Behavior change shouldn't feel like pulling teeth.

By understanding how you can change your habits without relying on willpower and without depending on a high level of motivation, your success rate will skyrocket.

The ability to stay lean 365 days out of the year has less to do with how much self-control you have and more to do with the health habits you practice regularly.

Change is not easy. I get that. But white-knuckling your way through is not the answer.

LIKE WHAT YOU DO

I see two primary issues in people who are trying to get in shape: They try to go too hard too fast, and they give up too soon.

You have to like what you're doing to keep it up consistently. Really, when you boil it all down, it's as simple as that.

If you enjoy your program, you're more likely to adhere to it. If you're consistent over the long term, it eventually pays off and you start to see the results you're after.

Put another way, the best fitness program for you is one that you can stick to.

Refusing to settle for anything less than the perfect diet and the optimal workout plan is an exercise in futility (no pun intended). Yes, in an ideal world, you'd never experience a hankering for added sugars and you'd crave broccoli and kale all the time. Wouldn't that be nice? Unfortunately, we're not wired that way.

The next best scenario, then, would be to find the intersection between what you as an individual are willing and able to do (meaning, what's practical for you) and what health behaviors will get you the results you want. This is the sweet spot.

Don't try to force a square peg (that's you!) into a round hole (a program you're not suited for). Rather than trying to make your life fit your nutrition and workout program, we'll flip that around: We'll make your nutrition and workouts fit your life.

When putting together any kind of fitness regimen, be sure to ask yourself this question: Is this program something I can see myself doing a year from now? The answer in almost all cases should be yes. If the answer is no, you may want to rethink your strategy.

With the right program, you can say goodbye to eight-item food lists, and you certainly should not expect to make working out your part-time job. You have a life to live, after all, and we're trying to enhance it, not detract from it.

IS THIS A FAT-LOSS PROGRAM?

This is not a fat-loss program per se, but by implementing the principles in this book, you'll learn how to make exercise and nutrition work in your favor. In the process, you'll get stronger and leaner, but more importantly, you'll change the way you think about fitness.

Nobody enjoys yo-yo dieting; it typically happens as a by-product of impatience and extreme methods. This is not you—at least, not anymore.

Be careful not to lose sight of the long-term goal, which should be to thrive in everyday life. That's not going to happen if you don't have the patience to use sustainable methods for your fitness. Losing body fat is nice, of course, but results will be fleeting unless you can first master your mindset.

I could easily offer you a fat-loss regimen and send you on your merry way, but doing that would be irresponsible of me. You'll learn about the basics of nutrition, and we'll cover the important guidelines to adhere to as you find the eating strategy that best works for you. You'll implement a sound resistance-training program to build strength and muscle, and you'll seamlessly meld all of this into your life.

I'm here to teach you how to become the captain of your own fitness ship. Eventually, you'll know how to navigate your journey on your own without needing my help or anyone else's. Then, my friend, my job will be done.

I'm going to show you how to eat, lift, and thrive.

THE "EAT, LIFT, THRIVE" MANTRA

"We're a community of women who eat for health and for enjoyment, lift heavy, and thrive in all aspects of our lives."

The "eat, lift, thrive" mantra was born organically, and it perfectly embodies what my brand is all about:

■ **Eat**: Learning about protein, carbohydrate, and fat is fine and dandy, but how does that all translate into real life? What do you do when you find yourself at Uncle Jon's Thanksgiving dinner staring at a delicious dish of homemade stuffing? When your month is booked solid with social engagements, how do you navigate all the food and alcohol without feeling remorse or guilt and without derailing your fitness goals? We cover that here.

■ **Lift**: Strength training is the fountain of youth. By building strength and increasing muscle mass, you improve not only your physical health but also your mental health. Yes, ladies, I'm talking to you! Exercise keeps you young; movement should be a way of life.

■ **Thrive**: Who cares that your training and nutrition regimen is pristine if you're unhappy and miserable and you've lost all your friends? I've been there, done that. And no thank you; I'm not interested in living that life anymore. How can you eat and exercise for your health and fitness goals and still live a full, rich life? It all starts in your head.

In this book, we'll first undergo a major overhaul of the mindset because, after all, unless the mind is in the right place, knowledge will not translate into application. We'll then cover nutrition and go over what I call the living-lean guidelines. Next, we'll review the eight movement patterns of strength training and learn how to build a better body. To wrap things up, you'll learn how to gauge and monitor your progress to become your own lifelong coach.

Let's get this show on the road.

PART

I

Reset Your Thinking

The first section of this book focuses on what I believe to be the most important aspect of your fitness journey: Your mindset.

Too often, people obsess over the minutiae of trying to find the perfect exercise regimen and the ideal fat-loss foods without taking the time to hone their mindset first. I made this mistake as well, once upon a time. In my mind, the mental aspect didn't matter; it was simply about trying harder and proudly making sacrifices left and right. I couldn't have been more wrong! Without my head in the right place, my quality of life quickly took a hit. I stopped enjoying my workouts, and I grew to hate my nutrition plan.

The details of a training and nutrition program are irrelevant if your mindset is not in the right place first. Conversely, if you can learn to become the master of your own mind, everything else becomes a cakewalk.

Chapter 1 begins by asking you to forget everything you thought you knew about fitness. I'll address some common psychology-related misconceptions about obtaining and maintaining results, discuss why it's beneficial not to rush the process, and talk about why you need to embrace sustainable methods.

Chapter 2 is all about embracing mistakes and learning from them to get better. You'll learn about why no single mistake is ever a big deal and how these errors offer an excellent opportunity for improvement.

Finally, chapter 3 discusses the importance of surrounding yourself with like-minded people (in person or virtual) who support your goals. I'll dive into one aspect of this journey you should always try to prioritize: quality of life.

Mastering your mindset isn't easy and may take some time, but I can assure you that the effort will be completely worth it. Let's begin.

CHAPTER 1

Forget What You Know

Every year when January 1 rolls around, millions of people around the world resolve to get lean and healthy—for real this time. Maybe you have a friend who has done this: She swears off all junk food, slashes her calories in half, and signs up for the most grueling boot camp classes available. Although it took years for the body fat to accumulate, she reasons that if she simply pushes hard enough for three short months, she can soon fit back into her skinny jeans and sport shredded abs.

At restaurants, she turns her nose up at the bread basket and instead orders a plate of sad, wilted lettuce with pieces of dry chicken breast. No dressing, of course, and she doesn't even think about adding croutons. Breakfast is half a cup of oatmeal, three egg whites, and two measly almonds; lunch might be steamed broccoli with white fish; and dinner is a protein shake. That's it? That's it.

In the gym, she throws herself to the wolves. Squats until she pukes. A thousand and one crunches. Lunges for days! Hours upon hours of mind-numbing jogging. The more fatigued she feels, the happier she is.

"Go hard or go home!" she yells.

Yet not even two months later, she has taken up residence on her couch again and is right back to a steady diet of egg rolls, pizza, and french fries. To add salt to the wound, she's not only undone all her progress but is now actually sitting about 10 pounds (4.5 kg) heavier than when she started.

Frustrated, she claps her hands together and resolves to do even better next time. It's just a matter of wanting it badly enough, she says, and she has to keep pushing through when the going gets tough, no matter what. So a 20-item food list gets further restricted to just 12 measly items, and she cranks up the ante on the cardio. *Ya gotta wanna!*

But time and time again, after one failed fat-loss cycle after another, she looks in the mirror and finds herself packing on more and more weight over time. In short, she's yo-yo dieting.

Does this sound fun, or good, for you? Do you think your friend feels successful and confident? Of course not.

People are good at weight loss; they're not so great at weight-loss maintenance (Kramer et al., 1989). This statement may not make much sense at first glance. Did she simply not try hard enough? Maybe she needed to perform a thousand and two crunches instead of a thousand and one. Why didn't she see immediate and lasting results?

When one of my clients, Morgan, first signed up with me, she was exasperated. She claimed to have tried every diet under the sun, yet her confidence was at an all-time low and her body weight at an all-time high. She said one line in particular to me that made me stop in my tracks: "Extremes are so easy; moderation is hard!"

There you have it. In a mere seven words, she had summed up our struggle with weight loss.

Over the past five years, I've worked with more than 1,000 fat-loss clients in some way, shape, or form. Most of them come to me to take over the reins of both their exercise and nutrition regimen, and I make it a point to address the mindset and behavioral aspects of their journeys as well. After all, I've come to learn that unless you have the right mental tools to succeed, all the training and diet knowledge in the world will be for naught.

An estimated 45 percent of our daily eating behaviors are governed by habit (Wood, Quinn, and Kashy 2002), meaning that a large portion of what and how much we eat occurs without much conscious thought. We all know what a habit is: An automatic behavior that occurs repeatedly in response to a specific context cue. This behavior can be anything from chewing gum during class to tying your shoelaces a certain way. And why do habits matter? Because they play a critical role in long-term behavior change. Understanding how they work and how we can use them to better our lives are key aspects that we'll circle back to later.

Let me enlighten you by addressing a few misconceptions.

■ **Myth 1: It's simply a matter of having enough willpower.** Willpower can be useful in many circumstances. It can prevent you from rolling your eyes in front of your parents when you're being lectured, it can keep you calm and collected when the idiot behind you at the movie theater won't stop kicking the back of your seat, and it can help you pass on the dessert menu at your favorite diner. In other words, its purpose is to help you do the right thing even when you want to do something else. But applying self-control feels fatiguing (Inzlicht, Berkman, and Elkins-Brown 2016), and if you use it enough throughout the day, eventually you'll cave (van Strien, Herman, and Verheijden 2014).

■ **Myth 2: The more you white-knuckle it, the better off you'll be**. A notion out there is that getting fit and healthy has to *feel* hard if you are to make meaningful progress; otherwise, you must be doing something wrong. The truth is, however, that the process should feel as easy as possible—in other words, struggle should be minimized. The less you struggle, the less energy you have to exert toward inhibiting unwanted desire and the more effective you will be at executing the target behaviors regularly (Galla and Duckworth 2015).

■ **Myth 3: If you're not going to go all out, then it's not worth doing at all**. We're impatient, and we don't like doing things halfway. If we're trying to get somewhere, we look for the fastest route possible, and most times we don't think of the long-term implications of our extreme behaviors. In a similar way, when we set ambitious fat-loss goals with unrealistic timelines, we probably do so when we're well fed, full of energy, and eager to shed the extra body fat. We assume that we'll continue to feel this way for the next three months. Crash dieting sounds like a good idea (for now), and pairing that with gut-wrenching workouts is even better! Unfortunately, we fail to appreciate just how difficult a given situation will be in the future when circumstances are different, a phenomenon known as the hot–cold empathy gap (Loewenstein 2005). We forget how unpleasant it is to feel tired, depleted, and hungry and how much harder it becomes to hit the gym six days a week. Suddenly, giving up seems like the easier, far more appealing thing to do.

All-or-nothing behaviors would be perfectly fine if we could sustain them year after year. But eventually something has to give.

SLOWER AND SUSTAINABLE IS BETTER

If we don't want to go all out and it's not about having an infinite supply of willpower, then how in the world do we change our habits and lifestyles for the better? We do it by making small, gradual changes to our everyday lives that don't feel so painful.

In other words, you not only have to like what you're doing but also have to be confident that what you're doing now is a behavior you can maintain for the long haul. The question that I pose to my clients when they consider adopting a behavior change is this: *Can you see yourself keeping this up for a year?* If the answer is yes, then they can go ahead and implement the behavior. If the answer is no, something needs to change.

If you've been living a sedentary lifestyle with zero formal exercise, then perhaps bumping up your physical activity to two days a week of weightlifting is a realistic place to begin. This plan is not extreme, no, but it's a start. And far more important, the regimen is probably one you can keep up week after week and month after month. Contrast this approach with trying to go from zero to hero overnight by signing up for every fitness class that you can cram into your schedule. Although at first you may brag that pumping away at the gym has practically become a part-time job (unpaid, mind you), chances are that you're eventually going to give out and find yourself right back at square one.

Instead of thinking only about the next few months, I encourage you to take a step back and consider where you want to be in six months, one year, and three years from now. Most of you probably won't be able to keep up six hard workouts a week indefinitely, but doing a couple of workouts a week may be something you can manage. How about cutting 300 calories out of your daily diet by slightly decreasing the portion sizes of your meal? Doing that probably won't hurt too much.

Those actions are sustainable behavior changes, and consistency is the name of the game.

Although seeing drastic results quickly is admittedly awe inspiring, I argue that it's far more respectable to get healthy and *stay* healthy. And ultimately, this is what we all want, isn't it—to quit the diet cycle at last, to maintain a lean and strong physique, and to feel good about ourselves? To accomplish these goals, we need a concrete game plan—one that isn't simply the flavor of the moment. We need to find something that'll stick for good.

First, start with small, bite-sized habits. Instead of going out for an hour-long walk every day, how about starting with 10-minute walks three days a week? Whatever you decide to do has to be manageable, not just today or this week, but indefinitely. The behavior goals should be easy, and ridiculously so. The point is to be able to execute the target habit regardless of how you're feeling and what else you have going on in your life. If you find that you can't keep up your habit consistently, it's probably still too big. Your habits should be three things: They should be small, they should be specific, and they should be meaningful so that they bring you closer to your goal. As you'll learn later, adherence to a nutrition program is the biggest determinant of lasting weight-loss success (Alhassan et al. 2008), so you should be prioritizing behaviors that you can adhere to day in and day out.

Next, make laziness work in your favor. Humans are inherently lazy (Selinger et al. 2015). By default, we choose the path of least resistance, and we want to conserve energy. Therefore, you need to adjust your environment and surroundings so that your laziness serves you rather than hinders you. If chocolate is your kryptonite, remove it from your home. If you can't do that, move it to the back of the highest shelf in your pantry behind the electric mixing bowl that you hardly use. That way, if you ever want to eat chocolate, you'll have to exert a whole lot of effort just to reach it, and you'll probably end up reaching for the banana sitting on your kitchen counter instead. This concept is known as *choice architecture* (Thorndike et al. 2012). To put it another way, you are making the healthier behavior the easier thing to do.

Finally, build positive momentum. Think about how discouraged you feel when you cave and down a pint of ice cream after vowing not to have any desserts for the entire month. Now think about how confident you feel when you successfully meet your goal of doing three air squats every time you use the bathroom. It's about *feeling* successful, no matter the size of the task at hand. Keeping momentum going is much easier, regardless of the pace. Having a string of successes can help build confidence and further motivate you to tackle bigger tasks later on.

Even if you master just two small habits per week, by the end of one year you'll have adopted 104 new habits that you didn't have before! Don't overlook the power of small steps that can accumulate over time.

HOW DELAYED GRATIFICATION SERVES YOU

Let's say you have a brownie sitting on a plate in front of you. As it so happens, you've got a serious sweet tooth. The thought of the sugar hitting your lips has you salivating in an instant. It's yours for the taking right this second, but I strike a deal with you. If you leave the treat untouched for the next 15 minutes while I'm out of the room, you can double the amount when I get back.

What do you do?

In the 1980s Walter Mischel conducted this very test with over 600 children between the ages of four and six using a marshmallow as the treat of choice (Mischel, Shoda, and Rodriguez 1989). The now-famous marshmallow experiment presented the young participants with a choice that tested their decision to have either one treat now or twice the reward after a short wait.

As you can probably imagine, the results were mixed. Some of the children pounced at the marshmallow as soon as the researcher left the room, whereas others actively employed distraction techniques, such as covering their eyes or turning their chairs away from the table to abstain from consuming the sweet treat.

OK, great. Mischel was able to show that even young children have the ability to practice delayed gratification, the ability to resist an immediate temptation in exchange for a greater reward after a time delay. Pretty neat, right?

The experiment didn't end there, though. The most significant findings of this study came in the follow-up on these same children more than 10 years later. Those who had successfully waited the 15 minutes for the second treat had higher SAT scores and were rated by their parents as being more attentive, competent, and intelligent. They were also better at resisting temptation and coping with stress. In short, the more skilled the children were at self-regulation, the better they performed in many aspects of life in their later years.

You can see delayed gratification paying dividends in your everyday life. If you abstain from checking your phone for an hour, you can finish your work faster and go home earlier. If you push back dinner with your friends by an hour, you can squeeze in your final workout of the week. If you resist touching your savings account long enough, you'll eventually have enough money to buy that hot sports car you've been eyeing.

You are absolutely allowed to inhale an entire chocolate cake in one sitting; technically, you're not breaking any laws. But if you practice self-regulation and limit yourself to just one slice, then next week you can come back for another slice with minimal ramifications to your waistline. You can opt to skip your afternoon postlunch cookie so that you can indulge in hot cocoa by the ice-skating rink later this evening without going overboard with your calories.

You'll notice that delayed gratification comes with a promise of a reward for waiting and then delivery of that reward. Everybody wins if you can just sit tight for a little while.

Delayed gratification is a skill that anyone can learn. The ability to practice discipline, rather than be impulsive all the time, is invaluable to success in any facet of life. Even if you think you're not that great at it now, you can improve this skill. Here are some methods to become better at waiting for a later reward:

■ **Stay distracted**. As Mischel and colleagues found during the marshmallow experiment, many of the children who successfully waited the 15 minutes without touching the first marshmallow did so by intentionally diverting their attention. They would turn their chairs away and focus their energies elsewhere for a time to obtain the prize of two marshmallows.

■ **Become part of a supportive community**. If you surround yourself with people who share a common goal and understand your struggles, you're far more likely to stick with the pursuit of a goal. You'll remember your reasons for starting your journey in the first place, you'll be able to celebrate your successes with others and find more meaning in your endeavor, and you'll be encouraged by others when you hit a speed bump.

Science Plug

I bring up Mischel's marshmallow experiment because it's considered the keystone study in the field of self-control. He uses the term *delayed gratification* throughout his paper, which is why we're using it here in this book. But *delay discounting* is considered the more empirical term, and it refers to the change in the perceived value of a reward according to its temporal proximity (Green, Fry, and Meyerson 1994). In other words, the further away in time a reward is, the less value it has. Delay discounting has been found to be associated with higher incidences of smoking (Bickel, Odum, and Madden 1999), drug dependence (Bickel and Marsch 2001), lower income and education (Reimers et al. 2009), obesity (Weller et al. 2008), and other life outcomes. In short, delay discounting—or delayed gratification—is a critical piece of the behavior equation, not only for mastering fitness but also for achieving overall life success.

■ **Make the tempting behavior the harder thing to do**. Put another way, if you make it more of a nuisance to do something, you're more likely to opt for an easier, alternative route. Commit yourself to showing up to the gym with your training partner; the desire to thwart the social pain that would result from your ditching the workout and letting your buddy down will motivate you to get up off the couch. Move the bowl of chocolates to the top shelf of the pantry or, better yet, remove it from your home altogether.

Fortunately, you're going to learn about all these concepts and more. In the coming chapters, you'll discover why it's important to get your mindset in the right place, and you'll gain the mental tools you'll need to succeed over the long haul. Before you roll your eyes and skip ahead to the nutrition and training sections of this book, hear me out.

I struggled in the first several years of my fitness career to practice what I preached: to lift weights regularly, to consume a high protein diet, to drink sufficient water, to tailor energy intake according to goals. On paper, these behaviors seemed like no-brainers, but I couldn't understand why simply *knowing* something didn't mean I'd be good at *doing* it. In other words, why were knowledge and application so far apart? Why did I self-sabotage by binging every few days, and why couldn't I maintain my body weight?

It didn't make sense to me for a long time, and I thought I was a failure. I believed, as coaches and colleagues told me at the time, that achieving success was simply a matter of trying hard enough. So after yet another nutrition screw-up, I'd dust myself off, slap my hands together, and vow that next time would be better if I could be stricter with myself. And like clockwork, three or four days later, I'd find myself back at square one.

Not until I realized that there was a crucial element not often talked about in the fitness equation did the lightbulb go off in my head. The training and nutrition program itself wasn't the problem; the issue was my mindset. It hit me that until I could get my mind in the right place, I'd continue spinning my wheels with my endeavors to improve my strength and physique.

The answer is not to try harder or to dig your heels more stubbornly into the ground. Rather than trying to force yourself through a brick wall, doesn't it make more sense to look around you and realize that walking around the wall would be far easier? This alternative is what mastering the mental aspect of the journey will be like.

You shouldn't have to feel like you're beating your body into submission. It's not normal to lie awake at night, stare at the ceiling, and wonder whether it's really supposed to feel this hard (the answer: It's not). You don't have to hate your meals or dread your workouts.

My job in the coming pages is to convince you to take things slowly, to be kinder to yourself, to embrace your mistakes, to focus on progress over perfection, and to navigate the middle ground. I get that it's a scary idea. But after many years of frustration and pain, aren't you ready for something a little different? Aren't you aching for a strategy, a lifestyle that you can enjoy while getting what you want out of your efforts in the kitchen and in the gym?

I'm here to teach you that and more. Get ready, because your life is about to change for the better.

ACTIONABLE ITEMS

- Embrace the smarter-not-harder route. Successful fitness isn't about white-knuckling your way to the finish line or going to extremes.
- Find behaviors that will both get you closer to where you want to be and be sustainable over long term. Ask yourself this: Can I keep up this behavior for a year?
- Start with small behavior changes, design for laziness, and build success momentum on your fitness journey.
- Delay gratification by staying distracted, becoming a part of a supportive community, and making the tempting behavior the harder thing to do.

CHAPTER 2

Failing Forward

I used to be deathly afraid of screwing up. In high school, I was a straight-A student. I prided myself on submitting my papers early, consistently beating my classmates on tests, and going above and beyond with every academic assignment. I woke up early and stayed up late to perfect academic assignments. I expected nothing less than the best from myself.

When it came to my fitness, circumstances were no different. As a varsity cross country athlete for seven years straight, I made it a point to log extra distance when everyone else was still sleeping, and I'd hang out in the weight room after practice to squeeze in my ab work. I'd spend my weekends running and swimming for several hours while my friends snoozed well past noon.

I believed that the harder I was on myself, the more successful I would be. And it worked for a while. I graduated at the top of my class and was admitted to my dream college. I slid easily into size-zero jeans and rocked a six-pack. My future seemed bright, and the rest of my life was bursting with potential.

Behind my pretty-on-paper life, however, it was a whole different story. In my pursuit of perfection, I alienated myself from my friends. In my hunger to be the best, I refused to help anyone else succeed, because I feared that the accomplishments of others would take away from mine. And I was so exhausted from trying to keep track of the 101 nutrition rules I'd imposed on myself that I'd find myself secretly binging on cookies and peanut butter a few nights a week.

I was miserable, but I didn't know any other way. I couldn't wrap my head around the fact that perfection was elusive and that failures were not necessarily catastrophic. I would launch into an ugly tirade with myself any time I didn't do as well as I'd expected on any given task, and I'd be discouraged by the smallest setback.

But, boy, was I wasting a lot of energy. Although I managed to do well for a time, the endeavor was exhausting and torturous. Most days, I was like a duck in a pond: I looked peaceful, serene, and composed above the water, but under the surface I was frantically paddling like crazy just to stay in the same damn place.

11

FIXED MINDSET VERSUS GROWTH MINDSET

I harbored a fixed mindset, which is the belief that traits and abilities are fixed and cannot be changed or improved (Dweck 2013). Whenever I violated any of my (admittedly arbitrary) diet rules, I interpreted my lapse as a sign that I simply was not destined to be in amazing shape. As I watched my friends laugh into their salads as though there was nothing else in the world they'd rather be eating, I wondered whether the fact that I had to choke down my tuna and egg whites meant that it wasn't in my genetics to be healthy. Because of this belief, I became consumed with looking the part. I pretended that sticking to the perfect diet came naturally to me. I talked nonstop about how much I enjoyed running (in fact, I was beginning to hate every minute) while secretly pigging out more and more on brownies, cookies, and candy. The more I stumbled, the more I tried to mask my true self. Unbeknownst to those around me, I ate and exercised the way I did not because I wanted to but because I felt trapped. The reality was that I was far from the picture of health—obsessing over what I couldn't eat, berating myself for not doing better, and becoming increasingly miserable with each passing day. In my pursuit of physical health, I neglected my well-being and quality of life.

Those with a fixed mindset actively avoid challenges and back down when they encounter an obstacle. They make excuses left and right about why they cannot do something. They play the victim. They balk at feedback, however well-intentioned, and do anything but exert effort.

Contrast them with people who have a growth mindset, which rests on the belief that ability, skill, and personal characteristics can be developed through dedicated effort. The growth mindset asks, "What can I learn from this so that I come back to do better next time?" whereas the fixed mindset proclaims, "Ah ha! Here is proof that I'm not cut out for this."

People with a growth mindset are all about self-improvement. When confronted with a setback, they actively work to improve their deficiencies and mistakes. They set out to learn and are constantly looking for opportunities for progress.

The work of Carol Dweck, a researcher at Stanford University, has been instrumental in highlighting how the mind can either impede change or open doors for a drastic transformation.

Interestingly, you may have a growth mindset in one area of your life and a fixed mindset in another area. For example, you might dedicate several hours per week honing your piano-playing skills with the hopes of one day becoming a world-class musician but, at the same time, shy away from algebra studies because mathematical concepts simply don't come naturally to you.

Consider how you think about your nutrition, exercise, and even your physical body. What kind of language do you use with yourself? You may notice that you're extremely defeatist and that when something goes awry—for example, when you accidentally dive into a box of donuts—you play the victim. Or perhaps when you realize one day that you can't zip up the dress that fit you three months ago, instead of sobbing into your pillow you immediately commit to scaling back your daily wine consumption.

The good news is that you can learn the growth mindset. Simply knowing about the two mindsets can allow you to recognize which way you tend to lean and then redirect your thinking. Whatever thoughts you harbor right now about your potential can be changed for the better.

You always have room for growth; you can always do something. You just have to believe it to be so.

OBSTACLES ARE A POSITIVE CHALLENGE

Imagine you've had a difficult day. You woke up to your dog puking all over your new carpet, you were pulled over and issued a ticket on the highway for texting while driving, and to top it all off, you received a less-than-stellar performance review at work. How would you respond?

If you have a fixed mindset, you'll likely throw a fit. You'll go on and on about how the world is unfair and how someone out there is obviously out to get you. You might say, "My life sucks," "Everyone has it better than I do," or "Of course, all these horrible things happen to me."

Client Profile: Kim S.

All my life, I thought I needed extreme willpower and absolute control to achieve my fitness goals. What I truly needed was to let go. I needed to change my mindset.

Growing up, I was always critical of my figure, and I wanted to change and fix it. After my first years in college, I was diagnosed with an eating disorder. It took nearly two years to repair most of the physical damage I did to my body, but the mental journey to a healthy mindset took much longer. For several years after my eating disorder, I struggled with anxiety and food fear, and I obsessively thought about my body and my plan for achieving the perfect look. Occasionally, the fear and anxiety diminished, but when I was stressed and tired, it came back. Eventually, I noticed I was spending more time and mental energy thinking and obsessing about food and my body than on all other areas of my life combined.

I joined Sohee's team in as an online client in January 2016. I was prescribed to eat more and work out less. Every day sirens screeched in my mind warning me to stop. Every day I thought I was losing control over my body. I cried, I got angry, and I questioned whether I was going the right things. I wanted to quit and go back to my old habits where I felt safe. But I dug deep, reminded myself that my old ways were not healthy or sustainable, and accepted the fact that change is uncomfortable. I stuck to my plan and, little by little, the obsessive thoughts that ran circles in my mind started to go away.

After I became flexible and open to mental and physical changes, I finally relaxed. When I relaxed, my fitness goals no longer seemed so daunting. For numbers' sake, in a year's time I went from lifting a combined total of 405 pounds (184 kg) 1RM for squat, bench, and deadlift to 600 pounds (272 kg) 1RM. I went from several hours of intense cardio a week to zero cardio. I eat almost 1,000 calories more a day, and I eat out three times a week minimum. I sleep through the night, and I think clearly. I weigh more, but I wear the exact same clothes I wore when I was 15 pounds (7 kg) lighter, which tells me that I've gained muscle mass and lost body fat. And, most important, I'm happy.

I expect more challenges in my fitness journey. There will be days when I will feel stuck, out of control, and I will struggle mentally. But I will continue to develop my positive mindset because I know that without a lasting mental improvement, there is no lasting physical improvement for me.

It's not that you're an inherently negative person. As long as life is going just the way you like it and you're receiving accolades left and right, you're probably a hoot to be around. But when you're faced with an obstacle you don't know how to cope with, you don't do so well.

In contrast, if you have a growth mindset, you might respond to the same day with the following statements: "I probably shouldn't leave my snacks out for the dog to get into when I'm not watching." "It's not safe to be texting and driving anyway—the cop taught me an important lesson." "My boss is right—I haven't been as focused at work lately. This is unlike me. I'll step it up and receive a better review next quarter."

Does this mean that I expect you to clap your hands together and do a backflip every time you get a C– on a midterm or your child does something in public that makes you feel like the world's worst parent? Should you celebrate downing a gallon of ice cream (3.8 L) when you were planning on the grilled chicken breast with steamed broccoli? Not quite. You're allowed to feel upset, and it's perfectly normal to feel distressed. The key difference is what you do with that disappointment. Do you turn a former setback into a future success?

Of course, people with a fixed mindset are not complete losers. In fact, they can succeed in life, but only as long as circumstances are moving along swimmingly in their favor. They want everything to be easy, because that is when they're happiest. Then they have the validation that they're looking for that they're naturally smart and capable.

Unfortunately, life does not occur in a vacuum, and we're constantly presented with challenges. You can be thankful that your beloved terrier only got an upset stomach from inhaling that chocolate bar and realize that the incident will help you become a better dog owner. Rather than wishing ill will on the police officer who issued you a ticket, you can be glad that nobody got hurt and take it as a wake-up call to be a more alert driver. And finally, you can be happy that your boss, although not thrilled with your work, is giving you an opportunity to redeem yourself and genuinely wants to see you thrive in your position.

Notice that these situations are unfortunate, but not catastrophic or devastating by any means. You'll hardly even remember these events three years from now, and when you approach them the right way, they can make you better.

You may be surprised at what you can accomplish if you take on obstacles as an opportunity to rise to the occasion.

NOTHING IS EVER UNFIXABLE

Twelve years ago, I suffered from anorexia and bulimia. In my darkest days, I was consuming nothing but a few sips of water and running 15 miles (24 km) on top of doing 5,000 crunches and 300 push-ups every single day. No, those are not typos. I was terrified of any food, and with my severely limited knowledge of nutrition, I mistakenly believed that ingesting anything with calories would mean that I would be fat for the remainder of my days. But twice a week, I would become so tormented that I would eat anything and everything I could get my hands on within the span of about two hours. I would make myself physically ill to the point of throwing up. I'd then spend the next three days trying to repent, so to speak, for the error of my ways.

Suffice it to say that I wasn't living a peaceful existence. I would spend every waking hour dreading my impending self-prescribed workout, and I couldn't get my mind off junk food. I believed that the harder I pushed myself and the more I suffered, the better results I would obtain. I was working harder, not smarter.

Now, a decade later, my world could not be more different. I no longer exercise to get sore and burn calories; I train to build strength and muscle. Instead of depriving myself of sustenance, I make it a point to consume a diet consisting primarily of nutrient-dense foods, and every now and then I enjoy a succulent treat. Better still, I have more muscle mass and less body fat than when I was running myself into the ground, and I feel a thousand times more energetic.

My experience is an extreme example of what can happen if you let your rigid thinking go too far. In my eyes back then, any deviance from my strict, arbitrary nutrition rules meant that I was doomed forever, and I thought that missing a workout meant that I'd surely wake up with a layer of extra body fat on my frame the next day. *If I eat this donut, it can never be undone. If I drink this milkshake, I'll be fat for life.* I was wracked with guilt, and I could never enjoy a single treat. I couldn't catch a break!

What I didn't understand back then was that nothing is ever unfixable. Just because I had a high-sugar meal for breakfast didn't mean that the rest of the day was shot; I could simply make my lunch more nutritious. Perhaps a chicken salad with extra veggies. Maybe a lean cut of steak with a baked potato. Now that I know better, I can do better.

The beauty of navigating your own fitness journey is that you have all the room in the world to make mistakes. You can try different methods and learn about what does and does not work for you. You have plenty of room for error to better refine your methods.

When it comes to exercise, of course, a horrific injury could have you sidelined for the remainder of your days. For that reason, erring on the side of caution is always a good idea. Execute proper form and avoid movements that induce pain. Otherwise, however, I embrace blunders and missteps because they serve as an invaluable learning opportunity.

"A moment on the lips, forever on the hips" is one of the most inaccurate and misleading quotations I've ever heard. It instills fear into people who believe that enjoying a slice of coconut cream pie means permanent doom and implies that they can never achieve redemption. This idea couldn't be further from the truth.

Yes, overindulgent eating today will probably mean that you'll be up a little on the scale tomorrow, and you may experience some temporary bloat. Oh well. The good news is that you're always just one meal away from making better choices and pulling your act together.

No single nutrition incident will do you in for good. I'm a fan of these missteps because they make for the best learning lessons. With some nonjudgmental reflection, you can figure out how and why that may have happened and come up with an actionable plan to prevent it from happening again in the future.

When you give yourself permission to let go of the need to be perfect, you'll find that you not only perform better but also see better results. We're not robots; we're humans. We're expected to make mistakes from time to time, and when we can practice compassion and bounce back quickly rather than wallow in disgust and pull the plug prematurely, we leave ample opportunity for improvement.

We may take two steps forward and one step back every now and then, but that sequence will beat two steps forward and two steps back any day.

When faced with a challenge, do you lean into the struggle, or do you throw in the towel?

After you train yourself to start thinking with a growth mindset, you'll view obstacles in a whole new light. One setback—in the kitchen, in the gym, or otherwise—does not make you a failure. You can always do something to get better.

EVERYTHING IS A LEARNING OPPORTUNITY

In 2015 popular NBC news anchor Brian Williams admitted to fabricating his role in a helicopter episode in Iraq (Wemple 2015). Until then, he seemed to have it all: He was the head of the news show and made frequent appearances on *Saturday Night Live* and the TV sitcom *30 Rock*. Millions of people trusted and respected him. Yet seemingly overnight, he lost all credibility with one made-up story.

He's far from the first journalist to lie. Mike Tobin of Fox News falsely claimed in 2011 that he'd been punched by a protestor (Judson n.d.). In 2013 ABC News chief White House correspondent Jonathan Karl lied about a Benghazi story. And for three straight years, *New Republic* reporter Stephen Glass published articles on events and people that never existed.

Most people would hear these stories and probably think that the culprits were nothing more than cunning, greedy professionals obsessed with making it to the top. But these people were likely crippled by the thought of being anything less than the best. They were trapped in the fixed mindset, and in a desperate attempt to look good and rise to eminence, they resorted to skipping the hard work and telling their own tall tales.

Those with a fixed mindset take shortcuts so that they can see faster results rather than take the time to lay a proper foundation for long-term success. They lie, cheat, and steal because they care more about looking smart and competent than acquiring the true skills needed to master their craft.

Don't be afraid to roll up your sleeves and do the dirty work. Experiencing a failure does not make you a failure. On the contrary, failing means that you're willing to put yourself out there and wade the waters of unfamiliar territory. That takes guts!

So you screwed up. What can you learn from it?

If you accidentally finished off the family-size bag of chips on your own while watching TV, you'll know next time to pour out a more reasonable portion size for yourself before getting comfortable on the couch. If you grazed throughout the day and couldn't feel satiated no matter what snacks you picked out, perhaps you should try increasing your protein intake and sitting down for a full-sized meal. If you failed on your squats today, you may want to watch your videos multiple times to see whether the problem was wonky form or too much weight so that you can correct the problem for next week.

Your beliefs about your potential and abilities have a powerful domino effect on your future behaviors and can determine whether you make moves to turn things around or continue on the path to self-destruction.

Let no mistake be in vain.

Learning to embrace your mistakes and get excited about your failures is easier said than done. You have to get outside your comfort zone and may have to undo several years, perhaps even decades, of believing that anything less than perfection is a waste of time.

Fortunately, you don't have to go at it alone, and in fact you shouldn't. This journey isn't meant to be taken solo.

In the next chapter, I'll discuss the importance of community. More specifically, you'll learn about how having a support system of people with shared interests and backgrounds will not only make this adventure a lot more enjoyable but also increase your adherence and thereby help you be successful over the long term.

ACTIONABLE ITEMS

- Embrace a growth mindset by seeing obstacles and mistakes as an opportunity to learn and become better.
- Reframe challenges by finding a positive takeaway.
- Don't despair about training and nutrition slipups; rarely is anything unfixable. You're always one meal away from reining yourself in again and making improvements and one workout away from executing exercises with better form and focus.

CHAPTER 3

You're Not Alone

As a female who lifts weights and prioritizes consuming a nutrient-dense diet, you'll likely find yourself among the minority in your school, work, or social setting. As much as I would love for it to be the case, being fitness-minded is not yet the norm.

Before dubbing yourself a lone wolf and embarking on this journey solo, I want you to understand that you don't need to go at this by yourself. You shouldn't, in fact. In this day and age, we are well connected to every corner of the globe. Even if you don't have peers in your vicinity who love to wax poetic about the latest protein-rich recipes or debate over proper deadlift form, you're only a few clicks away from finding a like-minded community online.

You may feel fully confident that you don't need a support system, but please hear me out. I spent my first several years lifting weights alone, celebrating gains alone, and fretting over my diet alone. I told myself that I was fine, that I didn't need any help, but the truth was that I was unbelievably lonely. I felt like I was living in a bubble, population one.

But my excitement rose to a whole new level when I became proactive about finding friends who loved fitness as much as I did. Who would have thought that I could discuss macronutrient breakdowns with a peer without her eyes glazing over? I never would have imagined that my training partner could be more delighted than I was when I set a deadlift personal record. Furthermore, I had people I could vent to or lean on for support when I became frustrated or discouraged with my progress.

One of the most memorable moments in my fitness career was when I was on stage at OCB Nationals competing for my bikini pro card. After weeks of diligent practice, I was finally strutting my stuff under the bright lights in 5-inch (12.5 cm) stilettos. As I struck one pose and smiled at the audience, my ears rang at the sound of my four girlfriends who had traveled all the way to Maryland just to root me on. They were all wearing my "Eat. Lift. Thrive." hoodies and shouting at the top of their lungs. When I finished my presentation and scurried backstage, my friends were waiting to give me bear hugs and take pictures. I had the biggest smile on my face, and my heart was full.

I flew back home that weekend with a pro card in my back pocket, but I was even more thrilled about the close-knit group of friends I had built. For someone who had started this journey completely alone, this meant the world to me.

I wasn't alone, and you shouldn't be, either. To thrive in your fitness adventures, surround yourself with people who have your back.

IMPORTANCE OF A SUPPORT GROUP

Many of my clients come to me with the goal of fat loss. We work closely together for a number of months, and I prescribe them a structured program based on their goals and their individual needs. They submit a check-in to me every two weeks, and then I make tweaks to their programs as necessary. It's all gravy.

Eventually, they reach their goal and really don't need me to guide them anymore. But when it comes time to part ways, they panic. They look out into the vast, open real world—sans coach!—and decide that maybe it'll be safer for them if they stick with me for a little while longer. So they tack on one more month. And then one more. Mind you, this is out of fear, not out of necessity. They erroneously believe that if they aren't accountable to someone at all times, they'll fall apart at the seams, somehow unlearn all the habits they've worked so hard to establish, and revert to their old ways.

But this concern is not warranted. You don't need to have a coach on your back at all times to succeed. You can stay accountable to your goals in a myriad of other ways, which may, in fact, be more effective.

Being a part of a like-minded community will be far better for you over the long haul than any single workout, diet, or seminar. Programs and facts are great, but they don't address the "how". You can know what to do, but you do not have a system in place for *how* to do it—not just once, but over and over until your behaviors become automatic habits. Information alone is meaningless if the knowledge does not translate into application. Having a support group helps solve that problem.

We are strongly influenced by the behaviors of those around us. Studies have shown this time and time again (Venkatesan 1966; Milgram, Bickman, and Berkowitz 1969). A 1990 study found that when more litter was scattered across the ground, 26.7 percent of subjects also littered, despite the fact that littering was harmful for the environment, compared with 10.7 percent of subjects who littered in a clean environment (Cialdini, Reno, and Kallgren 1990). The prevalence of littering increased because a littered surrounding had already been established as the normal state (known as the descriptive norm).

We can also see this pattern in eating behaviors. When dining with one other person, we tend to consume approximately 33 percent more calories (de Castro and Brewer 1992). With two others, that number rises to 47 percent, and with seven or more people, calorie consumption skyrockets to 96 percent more than when eating alone.

Whatever those in your immediate support group are doing, you will likely copy. This behavior reflects the power of social psychology. By and large, we want to fit in.

Of course, this principle can work in our favor if we are wise about the community we choose to get involved in, but it can just as equally harm us. Seek a community that has the same health interests and goals as you do and continue showing up.

Communities, however, are about far more than providing social context. They can help with habit formation (Wood and Neal 2007), encourage learning (Dragoni 2005), and increase self-efficacy (Hsu et al. 2007), which is a form of self-assessment. More specifically, self-efficacy refers to the evaluation of the self, and it affects motivation, and consequently, behavior (Bandura, 1982).

But simply bringing together a group of people who stand in the same place twiddling their thumbs is not sufficient. Technically, that group can qualify as a community, but the individuals must be working together to achieve a common goal.

When I say support group or community, you probably think of basement meetings on Wednesday evenings in your local neighborhood. That format certainly works, but many others mediums can work as well. Facebook groups, forums, e-mail chains, and text group chats are all examples of effective virtual communities. In real life, you have regular meet-ups for common interests such as hiking and cooking, and in recent years we've seen a rise in gym communities.

CrossFit takes the cake here (at least the Paleo kind). Regardless of your opinion on the exercise methodology, one thing cannot be denied: The CrossFit community is a force to be reckoned with. There's a reason why it's a profitable brand. Everyone knows one another by name, and more important, they cheer each other on with their daily Workout of the Day, or WODs. The WODs are excruciatingly difficult—there's no doubt about that—but thankfully you'll always have fellow athletes there to push you through and make it to the finish line.

I briefly joined CrossFit Magna, one of the bigger CrossFit boxes in the Phoenix metropolitan area. The owner, Brian Kunitzer, was kind enough to grant me access to his facility during open gym hours to perform my personal powerlifting workouts. Watching the gym members show up day after day, and more surprisingly, mingle both before and after their workouts to spend time together, was truly inspiring. You don't see this in a commercial gym. You don't see this in most gyms, period.

I'm not here to tout the life-changing wonders of CrossFit per se. Rather, I want to highlight the aspects of community that they do incredibly well.

CrossFit is about more than just the workouts, whereby individuals are brought together by a shared suffering. They spend time together outside the gym, attend each other's graduations, and are even in one another's weddings as groomsmen and bridesmaids. In November 2014, when the CrossFit Magna facility upgraded from a 2,200-square foot (204 sq. m) space to a location five times larger than its original size, the move took only two days. How? Dozens of members showed up with their trailers and trucks and donated their time and energy to help transport equipment. They received no financial incentive, no compensation, no membership discounts—none of that. What was in it for them? "They're proud of this space," reports Brian. "This is their own."

If that's not a community, I don't know what is.

McMillan and Chavis (1986) take it one step further in their definition of what makes up a community.

First, you need membership, a feeling that you've invested to become a member of a group and consequently feel like you belong (Aronson and Mills 1959). Such a membership provides boundaries, which promote a sense of emotional security and safety.

Next is influence, and this goes in both directions: The individuals must contribute to the group or must have already contributed in some capacity, and, conversely, the group must be able to influence its members.

The third element is integration and fulfillment of needs—reinforcement, in other words. The group must fulfill the members' needs, provide rewards that reinforce the community (status, success, capabilities), share individual values, and meet other people's needs while meeting their own.

Finally, a community must have a shared emotional connection. The members must have not only common interests and backgrounds but also positive connections with one another in some way.

You'll notice that the term *community* is broadly defined. A proper community can come in myriad forms, whether it is in person or online. Here's an example of how you can find yourself a group that fulfills all these requirements.

Through social media channels, you happen to connect with a handful of other women who love fitness as much as you do. You all enjoy lifting weights, and you prioritize your health by getting sufficient sleep, managing your stress levels, and cooking nutrient-dense meals regularly. You're thrilled to learn that their idea of a fun Friday night is spending the evening at the gym with no time constraints—and you thought you were the only one! After a bit of back and forth, you decide to reach out to everyone in a group text and invite them over to your garage gym for a monthly get-together. Even though some women live a few hours away, you quickly become a tight-knit group of fitness chicks. Eventually, you even have T-shirts made exclusively for the women in the group, and you're proud to consider yourself a member of this newfound community.

Why does this work well? This group of weightlifting women has everything it needs to become a powerful community with potential to grow: membership, in which some people clearly belong and others do not; influence, in which the women can support each other by providing accountability, sharing recipes, spotting each other at the gym, and bringing together the individuals through a common interest; and fulfillment of needs, in which the women can relate to each other's struggles, bond over personal victories under the barbell, and lament the lack of nutrient-dense options at the local buffet.

Good communities are powerful because they can make it harder *not* to do the right thing. If you miss a practice, other members will notice and will get on your back about your failure to show. If you don't submit your weekly check-in, you can bet that someone will be popping in to see how you're doing.

And it's not just about showing up. Communities provide a safe space for people to make mistakes, learn from the process, and keep going. Members pool their collective experience and pull out the tools they keep in their back pockets to offer support. Giving up is a lot harder when you have a whole crowd of people urging you to keep going.

Lasting behavior change does not occur in a bubble. Pay attention to the people you choose to surround yourself with. If you're not a part of a sound community just yet, I encourage you to do some digging now to find local or online communities you can connect with. Check out the actionable items list at the end of this chapter for suggestions to get started.

QUALITY OF LIFE ABOVE ALL

Nine months after I first learned how to lift weights, I was catapulted into the college world as a doe-eyed freshman. I was eager to enroll in a dozen different classes and make new friends, of course, but at the time I was more concerned with doggedly adhering to my fitness regimen. I'd been working throughout the summer to get stronger and lose body fat in an effort to obtain the look of a figure competitor. In hindsight, I was already incredibly petite—standing 5 feet, 2 inches (157.5 cm) and weighing 102 pounds (46 kg)—and was reaching the point of having to put in more and more work for increasingly diminishing returns. I turned a blind eye to a plethora of blatant red flags in my pursuit of what I considered the perfect physique. I became crabby, started avoiding social events out of fear of deviating from my program, and was having increasing trouble adhering to my strict meal plan.

As most college freshmen are wont to do, I initially stuck with my fellow classmates as we explored the unfamiliar campus together. We ate our meals at the same table, walked to class together, and helped each other through problem sets.

As the months wore on, however, I found myself withdrawing from my well-meaning friends. I made it a point to get to bed extra early so that I could be at the gym at 6 a.m. when the doors opened (and yes, this meant that I'd wake up at 5:30 a.m. on the dot). I ate more of my meals alone so that I could avoid explaining why I was choking down a dozen egg whites in one sitting. I sat alone in my room on the weekends as everyone else attended frat parties and went out to restaurants because I was terrified of deviating from my fitness program. Eventually, the invitations to hang out dwindled down to none, and I spent most of my time isolated in my own little world.

Truth be told, I thought I was better than everyone else for living this life. Oh, the sacrifice! I looked down on my peers for daring to sleep in past noon, and I judged them for scarfing down french fries for dinner. I was horrified that they would even consider helping themselves to a scoop of ice cream on a sunny Saturday afternoon. I believed that my regimen was what it took to be healthy, all the while completely missing the irony of the situation.

I had it completely backward.

Not until the end of that school year did I look around one day to realize that not only did I have no social life whatsoever, but I was unhappy. In my obsession to be fit, I had completely neglected my well-being.

Could you really blame me, though, for believing that leaner physiques will solve all of life's problems and lead to pure bliss?

Take a glance around at the images we're bombarded with. We have rail-thin models seemingly living the life of their dreams without a care in the world. Those with ripped abs and curves in all the right places are the object of admiration of thousands, if not millions, of men and women alike.

On social media, practically all we see are posts of fitness celebrities calling themselves role models while flaunting their bodies in tiny pieces of cloth that are hanging on for dear life. Never mind that they'd just spent the last 20 minutes trying to find the perfect lighting and just the right angle and body contortion to capture their physique in the most flattering manner—they're real, authentic people who just like to work out and eat well! *Please like my photo! Please envy my existence!* They brag about the gut-wrenching sacrifices they have to make to look the way they do. They're up at 5 a.m., eating dry chicken breast and broccoli for Thanksgiving dinner, spending upward of four hours at a time at the gym. But they're *happy*, so it's all OK.

Wow, we think to ourselves. *If only I could just drop these last 10 pounds (4.5 kg) of body fat, then my life will surely be as great as theirs is.*

All these behaviors rest on the following premise: She is lean; therefore, she is happy.

But that's not what matters. Achieving a fit, athletic, and lean physique certainly takes dedicated work, but at what point does the pursuit of a bootylicious derriere no longer justify the sacrifices being made?

That question never even crossed my mind until a few years ago. Cost? What cost? I'm here to get a rockin' body. What bad could possibly come out of that?

I was naive and didn't recognize that my quest to become the epitome of health led me down the opposite path. Why? Because I focused only on the physical, aesthetic aspect of fitness and neglected everything else.

At every point along the way, consider how your current fitness program is affecting the following:

- Energy level
- Mood
- Libido
- Stress
- Sleep
- Relationships
- Work

Obviously, you need to compromise to some degree. If you're going to start spending a handful of hours at the gym per week, that time has to come from somewhere. And when you are in a caloric deficit, it's normal for energy, mood, and libido to take a mild dip. But don't stubbornly forge ahead with your fitness goals if red flags are signaling you to hit the brakes.

An exercise and nutrition program may look great on paper, but if you're not feeling so hot and your regimen is negatively affecting relationships with your loved ones, I would seriously consider changing course. It's not worth it.

The purpose of fitness should be to enhance, not take away from, your quality of life. Don't forget that. Although participating in a bodybuilding competition or reaching your fat-loss goal in one go can be admirable, you need to consider the toll it could take on your physical, mental, and emotional health. If you become nasty tempered from eating at a caloric deficit for too long, what have you really gained? If you take home the first-place trophy but you've alienated yourself from your friends in the process, have you really won?

Rather than striving to look a certain way, you want to *feel* a certain way—strong, healthy, and full of energy. So instead of bending over backward to accommodate a fitness program, find the nutrition and exercise strategy that fits your life while still getting you to your goal.

Just because you can keep pushing the gas pedal on a fitness regimen doesn't mean you should. Set aside your ego and pay attention to the warning signs. How are your energy levels? Are you still pleasant to be around? Do you find yourself getting into petty fights? Do you dread your workouts? Do you hate the way you eat? Know thyself.

Never get so busy building a body that you forget to make a life.

In part II, we'll transition to discussing nutrition. After going over the fundamentals of protein, carbohydrate, and fat, I'll walk you through my living-lean guidelines, which are my recommended strategies to eat in a way that will fuel your body and complement your physique. Most important, you'll learn how to dominate your diet without having to resort to extremes. You'll become the master of moderation, and you'll effortlessly eat your way to some extraordinary, lasting results.

ACTIONABLE ITEMS

- Make a list of the types of groups and social settings in which you find yourself most comfortable. Do you typically spend most of your time interacting with others in Facebook groups, or do you have an e-mail chain with your friends? Do you thrive in an in-person setting, getting to know others face to face? That's the type of community you should seek.

- Online or in person, become part of a community of people with shared interests to help you in your fitness endeavors. Whether you're a new mom trying to get back into shape, a college student looking for peers who prioritize their health, or a 20-something living in a small town where female weightlifters are unheard of, find your tribe and get involved.

- Can you think of people in your life who would be willing either to join you on your fitness journey or to support your efforts? Recruit their involvement.

- Keep a pulse on your quality of life every step of the way. Pay attention to how your energy levels, mood, libido, stress, sleep, relationships, and work become affected by your quest to sculpt your body and become healthier. Hit the brakes or scale back when the results you're striving for are no longer worth the sacrifices you're making.

PART

II

Eat

If you think you need a quick refresher course on nutrition or if you're completely confused about where to begin, I recommend starting with chapter 4. I won't be going into comprehensive detail about every single micronutrient, but I want to make sure you get the gist of what is and is not important.

Then I'll walk you through my seven living-lean guidelines in chapter 5. Keep in mind that these guidelines are, by definition, not etched in stone. You should try to adhere to these principles most of the time, although deviations every now and then are acceptable and a part of living life.

Finally, chapter 6 teaches you how to tie together all the nutrition tools to mindlessly eat better and to make your diet fit your life (rather than the other way around!).

The beauty of my guidelines is that regardless of any dietary restrictions or food preferences you have, you'll be able to apply them to your own daily life. Whether you have an irregular work schedule that leaves you eating at odd hours or you are deathly allergic to eggs doesn't matter. I've intentionally left many parts open-ended because I don't know you personally and therefore can't tell you exactly what you need.

You know yourself best. With a little bit of introspection and digging, you'll be able to tailor my suggestions to fit your unique needs.

CHAPTER 4

Nutrition Basics

Most nutrition books present a long list of rules to follow. Eat this, not that; make sure to stir some magic oils into your coffee every morning to prompt the fat-burning process; consume carbohydrate only between the hours of 8:03 a.m. and 2:04 p.m., not a minute longer!

Before you dive straight into the latest fad diet and get caught up in all the hype, keep in mind that most of the time, that's all it is: hype.

It all seems overwhelming and confusing sometimes, doesn't it? Moreover, how often have you successfully followed through on a new trend and seen lasting results? I'm guessing that, because you're here now, the answer is never.

I fell for all of it, too, once upon a time. I drank skim milk instead of whole because I thought that consuming dietary fat would add to my waistline. I avoided french fries like the plague because they weren't considered clean enough. I spent hundreds of dollars on fat burners. I rushed home from the gym after my workout to get in my postworkout meal within the supposed 45-minute anabolic window, and I wailed in defeat if it was minute 47 by the time I took my first bite of food.

It seemed like a whole lot of work, let me tell you that. And to be honest, I felt like a martyr, making sacrifices left and right in the name of health and fitness. I was bending over backward and jumping through hoops chasing the elusive fat-loss carrot that I couldn't seem to grasp despite my painstaking efforts.

I reckoned that perhaps I was failing because I was consuming a 30 percent protein diet and needed to bump that up to 40 percent. I wondered whether eating spinach instead of broccoli would help me see better results. But I craved those french fries. And boy, did I want that ice cream sometimes.

None of it made sense to me. I felt that I was hurting a whole lot without much to show for it. To make matters worse, I watched in simultaneous horror and confusion as my thin friends joyfully consumed late-night churros and bonded over chicken nuggets every now and then. Didn't they know they weren't supposed to eat those foods? Why didn't they feel any remorse? Yet year after year, they stayed lean while I struggled to maintain a steady body weight.

It seemed so effortless to them and unfairly difficult for me. Was it purely genetics? Did they have some secret supplement that I was not privy to? Did they simply have more willpower than I did?

Thankfully, I know better now. I was missing the forest for the trees.

NUTRITION PYRAMID

Before we delve into how you can make nutrition fit your life and learn to eat your way to a slimmer, stronger you, you need to understand the hierarchy of nutrition. Not all elements of nutrition are created equal. Some aspects of what and how you eat will make a bigger difference in both your physique development and health than others. After you understand what facets hold greater weight, you'll be better equipped to channel your energies into seeing the changes you want.

Think of the various elements of nutrition like a pyramid. At the bottom are what I consider the big rocks. You should concern yourself with and master these first before worrying about the smaller pebbles at the top. In other words, focus on the things that matter the most before obsessing over the things that make only a smattering of difference.

We'll go over them in order of importance.

CALORIES

In the fall of 2014 I was getting ready for my national-level bikini show. For those unfamiliar with the bodybuilding world, bikini is one of several divisions in which women can compete. As a competitor, you are judged on both your looks (body-fat level, muscle symmetry, hair, makeup, tan) and your presentation (posing routine, walk, overall poise and grace). Many competitors undergo several months of a regimented training and diet program to shed body fat and build muscle in the right places so that they can step on stage looking the part.

The norm in the bodybuilding world is for competitors to adhere to a strict meal plan with a 12-item food list, and they'll go months and months without consuming any added sugars. Many even abstain from fruits, dairy, and any fat sources because they mistakenly believe that these foods will impede fat-loss efforts.

For this particular prep, I decided to do something unconventional: I fit a full-sized Snickers bar into my nutrition program. I ate a Snickers not just one time, but every single day for 70 consecutive days leading into the competition.

I lost 5 pounds (2.3 kg) of body fat and 2 inches (5 cm) off my waist in a six-week timespan. I came in at my leanest and, coincidentally, my best and most polished look, and I took home the first-place trophy in my height class, earning my pro card as an IFPA all-natural bikini competitor. That result was pretty sweet (no pun intended).

Before you ask, yes, I did get tired of eating the same treat every day for 10 weeks straight, and yes, I was glad to be done when D-day rolled around. But I took this unusual approach to drive home a point that I believed people needed to understand: If you control your overall calorie intake and consume sufficient protein, you can shed body fat while consuming a little bit of junk food.

This experiment was inspired by Dr. Mark Haubs, the man behind the infamous Twinkie diet. In 2010 the Kansas State University human nutrition professor embarked on a 10-week diet in which two-thirds of his 1,800 daily calories came from junk food such as Twinkies, Oreos, and sugary cereals (Park 2010). He lost 27 pounds (12 kg) and, perhaps more surprisingly, his low-density lipoprotein levels (the bad cholesterol) dropped by 20 percent while his high-density lipoprotein levels (the good cholesterol) increased by 20 percent. This outcome flew in the face of what we thought we knew about junk food—we believed that junk was inherently fattening. Dr. Haubs showed that this was not the case and that a consistent caloric deficit was what allowed him to shed body weight.

At the bottom of the nutrition pyramid, you have the most important component, which is your total calorie intake. A calorie is the amount of energy needed to raise the temperature of 1 gram of water by 1 degree Celsius; a kilocalorie, or Calorie, is the equivalent of 1,000 calories. The latter is what we use to discuss the nutritional value of food, but in colloquial terms, we typically don't capitalize the C. So when we say that a donut has 250 calories, we really mean 250 Calories.

Your energy balance—how much energy you consume versus how much you expend—determines whether you lose weight, maintain weight, or gain weight. Although many variables go into this equation, in general, it is a function of how much you eat through your daily diet in relation to how many calories you burn off through the thermic effect of food, nonexercise activity thermogenesis (NEAT), formal physical activity, and more.

Don't let this information overwhelm you. All this is saying is that to lose weight, you must burn off more energy than you take in, and to gain weight, the inverse holds true.

Finding the right energy balance for your goal is by far the most important piece of the nutrition equation. It's not about avoiding the egg yolk or replacing donuts with sweet potatoes or swearing off pizza forever, so don't get caught up in the eat-this-not-that craze.

The main reason that junk food tends to get a bad rap, aside from its admittedly dismal nutritional value, is that it's typically calorie dense compared with fruits, vegetables, and other wholesome, minimally processed foods. An apple, for example, may have 90 calories, whereas an equal-sized slice of cake may pack triple the calorie punch. And because these high-fat, high-sugar treats tend to be far more palatable, we tend to consume more. When we consume more, we ingest extra calories, which over time can add to our waistlines.

It's easy for people to reason that cakes, cookies, pizza, and chips are necessarily evil and that one bite of any of these foods will have your fat cells multiplying uncontrollably. But don't confuse correlation with causation. There are no magic fat-loss foods, just as there are no inherently fat-gaining foods.

Does this mean that I'm giving you the green light to consume nothing but donuts all day long? Not quite. Macronutrients come into play here.

MACRONUTRIENTS

After calories come the three macronutrients: protein, carbohydrate, and fat. Your body requires these nutrients in large quantities.

The foods you consume consist of various combinations of macronutrients. Some foods, such as meats and poultry, are dominant in one macronutrient, but most foods contain a mix of all three macronutrients.

You may have heard the term *counting macros*. This term refers to tracking the number of grams of protein, carbohydrate, and fat you consume during an entire day's worth of eating, usually with the intent on meeting a prescribed set of macronutrient numbers. People are increasingly using this method instead of simply counting calories.

Calories and macronutrients are necessarily related. One gram of protein contains 4 calories, 1 gram of carbohydrate contains 4 calories, and 1 gram of fat contains 9 calories. If you consume 100 grams of protein, 150 grams of carbohydrate, and 60 grams of fat in one day, a little bit of math will yield your total calorie intake:

$$(100 \text{ grams protein} \times 4 \text{ calories/gram}) + (150 \text{ grams carbohydrate} \times 4 \text{ calories/gram})$$
$$+ 60 \text{ grams fat} \times 9 \text{ calories/gram}) = 400 \text{ calories} + 600 \text{ calories} +$$
$$540 \text{ calories} = 1{,}540 \text{ total calories}$$

Being mindful of not only your overall calories but also the macronutrient breakdown of your daily diet can be important in ensuring that you are consuming enough of the right nutrients.

Protein

At a fundamental level, dietary protein is important for catalyzing biochemical reactions, aiding in DNA repair, maintaining the structural and functional integrity of cells, and more. It can be found in all of your body's living cells. That's all great, but what about its application to fitness buffs?

Evidence suggests that protein increases thermogenesis, or the energy required to digest food, and provides the most satiety of all the macronutrients (Halton and Hu 2004). This aspect is great from a fat-loss standpoint. In addition, consuming a large amount of protein coupled with consistent exercise improves body composition when in a caloric deficit—more specifically, body fat is lost and lean mass is largely preserved (Layman et al. 2005).

Contrary to popular belief, high protein intake has not been found to be harmful in healthy people (Martin, Armstrong, and Rodriguez 2005). In fact, research indicates that active, resistance-training people have protein requirements well above the recommended dietary allowance (RDA) of 0.8 grams of protein per kilogram of bodyweight to aid in muscle repair and adaptation to exercise stimulus (Phillips and Van Loon 2011). Consuming up to 2 grams of protein per kilogram of body weight per day may be beneficial for ambitious body composition and performance goals.

For the sake of simplicity, we can say that 1 gram of protein per pound (2.2 g per kg) of lean body mass is the general recommendation for most healthy individuals. You can scale up to 1 gram of protein per pound of total body weight if you're highly active, but this is a good starting point, especially for those of you starting out with higher body fat percentages.

Protein can come from both animal and plant sources. Meats, poultry, fish, eggs, and dairy products are considered complete proteins because they contain all the essential amino acids (EAAs) in the appropriate amounts. Most plant sources tend to be incomplete, meaning that they lack one or more of the essential amino acids. Therefore, a variety of plant-based sources must be consumed to obtain all the EAAs.

Here is a sampling of foods that consist predominantly of protein: steak, beef, pork, chicken, turkey, bison, ostrich, fish, cottage cheese, milk, Greek yogurt, protein powder, lentils, edamame, tofu, quinoa (table 4.1).

Carbohydrate

Technically, we can live without carbohydrates, or carbs for short. Our bodies will be just fine. But that doesn't mean that doing so will be pleasurable for us or will give us the energy levels we need to function at maximum capacity. Life is more fun with carbohydrate.

Table 4.1   High-Protein Foods

Protein source	Serving size	Calorie content	Protein content
Top sirloin steak, cooked	3 oz	140 kcal	25 g
96% lean ground beef, cooked	3 oz	139 kcal	22 g
Pork tenderloin, cooked	3 oz	131 kcal	23 g
Chicken breast, cooked	3 oz	134 kcal	25 g
Turkey breast, cooked	3 oz	125 kcal	26 g
Bison, cooked	3 oz	152 kcal	22 g
Ostrich, cooked	3 oz	146 kcal	22 g
Halibut, cooked	3 oz	97 kcal	20 g
Low-fat cottage cheese	3 oz	73 kcal	10 g
Low-fat milk	1 cup (approx. 245 g)	102 kcal	8 g
Fat-free Greek yogurt	1 container (approx. 170 g)	100 kcal	18 g
Protein powder	1 scoop (approx. 32 g)	130 kcal	25 g
Lentils, cooked	1 cup (approx. 200 g)	220 kcal	17 g
Edamame, cooked	1 cup (approx. 155 g)	189 kcal	17 g
Tofu, firm	1/2 cup (approx. 126 g)	88 kcal	10 g
Quinoa, cooked	1 cup (approx. 185 g)	222 kcal	8 g

Carbohydrate has been given a bad rap over the years. Demonizing foods such as breads and muffins that contain simple carbohydrates is easy because they tend to be devoid of quality nutrients. But we can't forget about the hierarchy of nutrition. All types of carbohydrate can be worked into a moderate nutrition program without derailing progress as long as you control for total calories.

As with just about anything, I don't take an extreme stance. And, of course, my primary purpose is to provide you with the tools you need to determine what intake is most appropriate for you.

Carbohydrate is the body's primary energy source, so in general, the more physically active you are, the more carbohydrate you should consume. You should also pay attention, however, to how you feel physically and mentally after consuming a carbohydrate-heavy meal. Some people feel highly energized, whereas others become lethargic, so you should adjust your intake accordingly.

I recommend a moderate carbohydrate intake to begin if you're not sure how much to consume. This means the portion of carbohydrate you should consume per meal should be roughly the size of your fist. You'll have to use some trial and error to find the amount that allows you to feel your best and perform well in the gym while working toward your fitness goal.

These carbohydrate-dominant foods serve as a starting point to give you an idea of where to get this macronutrient: white potato, sweet potato, white rice, brown rice, couscous, oats, squash, bread, cereal, fruit, and vegetables (table 4.2).

Table 4.2 High-Carbohydrate Foods

Carbohydrate source	Serving size	Calorie content	Carbohydrate content
White potato, cooked	1 cup (approx. 150 g)	116 kcal	27 g
Sweet potato, cooked	1 cup (approx. 133 g)	114 kcal	41 g
White rice, cooked	1 cup (approx. 158 g)	206 kcal	44 g
Brown rice, cooked	1 cup (approx. 195 g)	216 kcal	45 g
Couscous, cooked	1 cup (approx. 157 g)	176 kcal	36 g
Oats, dry	1 cup (approx. 81 g)	307 kcal	55 g
Yellow squash, cooked	1 cup (approx. 180 g)	36 kcal	8 g
White bread	1 slice	69 kcal	13 g
Kellogg's Frosted Flakes	1 cup (approx. 41 g)	151 kcal	37 g
Apple	1 medium	72 kcal	19 g
Broccoli	1 cup (approx. 91 g)	30 kcal	11 g

Fat

Fat is delicious—let's just get that out of the way first. And on top of being delicious, it can and should be incorporated as part of a normal healthy diet. Dietary fat is crucial for regular hormone function (particularly testosterone production) and helps improve blood lipids and reduce cardiovascular disease risk.

Fat is the most calorically dense macronutrient of the three, clocking in at nine calories per gram. But before you toss out your egg yolks and steer clear of added oils, keep in mind that we're not here to demonize any foods. Rather, we're learning to navigate the multiple food decisions we face on any given day. High-fat foods also tend to be highly palatable, so yes, we have to be mindful of how much we consume lest the calories skyrocket. A moderate intake, however, can help increase satiety through hormones such as cholecystokinin, peptide YY, and glucagon-like peptide-1, as well as decrease gastric emptying so that you feel full for a longer time.

You may be wondering about saturated fat, unsaturated fat, and trans fat. Which types are good for your health, and which should you steer clear from?

Without turning this into a nutrition textbook, here's what you need to know. Saturated fat is found in many animal-based fat sources, such as dairy (butter, cream, milk, cheese) and meat (fatty cuts of beef, lamb, and pork and processed meats such as sausage and salami). For a long time, people believed that saturated fat was bad for your health and caused heart disease. Even as recently as 2010, the United States Department of Agriculture (USDA) recommended that saturated fat make up a measly 10 percent or less of daily total calories (USDA and UDHHS). But studies have since concluded that the evidence is insufficient to associate dietary saturated fat intake with cardiovascular disease (Siri-Tarino et al. 2010), so we don't need to be afraid of consuming fat.

Unsaturated fat can be found in plant sources including olives, nuts, and seeds and is present as well in fish. Oils, such as olive oil, also fall into this category. Unsaturated fat is considered the healthy fat because it lowers plasma total and low-density-lipoprotein cholesterol levels (Howell et al. 1997).

The reputation of trans fatty acid has taken quite the beating over the years because of its contribution to increased coronary heart disease risk (Mozaffarian and Clarke 2009).

Table 4.3 High-Fat Foods

Fat source	Serving size	Calorie content	Fat content	Saturated fat	Unsaturated fat
Olive oil	1 Tbsp	119 kcal	14 g	2 g	12 g
Butter	1 Tbsp	102 kcal	12 g	7 g	3 g
Walnuts	1 oz	186 kcal	19 g	2 g	16 g
Pumpkin seeds	1/2 oz	82 kcal	7 g	1 g	5 g
Cheddar cheese	1 oz	114 kcal	9 g	6 g	3 g
Whole egg, large	1 egg	72 kcal	5 g	2 g	3 g
California avocado	1/2 avocado	218 kcal	10 g	1 g	8 g
Whole milk	1 cup	149 kcal	8 g	5 g	2 g
Heavy cream	1 Tbsp	51 kcal	6 g	3 g	2 g

Your Questions Answered

Q: Shouldn't I be concerned with the specific grams of protein, carbohydrate, and fat I'm consuming?

A: I won't list a specific breakdown of macronutrients because doing so goes against what we're about to learn, which is to eat without obsessing over numbers. I do recommend, however, that you pay attention to food labels and have at least a general awareness of approximately how much protein, carbohydrate, and fat are in what you're eating. If you want to see a food database, www.ChooseMyPlate.gov is a reliable resource.

Chances are that you've probably been told to avoid it like the plague, which is unfortunate because it can be found in many of your favorite packaged foods, including donuts, cakes, and cookies. What you probably don't know is that naturally occurring forms of trans fat are found in meat and dairy (Chardigny et al. 2008) and a form of trans fat called vaccenic acid may actually lower coronary heart disease risk. Moreover, to date, no research on humans has established a relationship between trans fatty acid and body composition, so for now, we can say that trans fat is fine to consume in moderation.

In terms of serving sizes, use your thumb as a guide.

Here are some sources of fat-dominant foods: oils, butter, nuts, seeds, cheese, whole eggs, avocados, whole milk, cream (table 4.3).

MICRONUTRIENTS

Next in the nutrition hierarchy are micronutrients, the vitamins and minerals that the body requires in minute quantities. Although we require only miniscule amounts of these nutrients—typically to the tune of milligrams or less—covering our nutritional bases can make a big difference in energy levels, mental alertness, physical performance, and more.

When people talk about some foods being more nutrient-dense than others, they're referring to the micronutrient content of said foods. For example, they may argue that a bowl of brown rice has a far better nutritional profile than a sugar-glazed donut—and to be fair, within that one isolated meal, they would be correct. No one's going to claim that a donut is chock full of quality micronutrients. But as we'll learn, diets should be assessed as a whole and within proper context.

Micronutrients can be categorized into minerals, which are inorganic, and vitamins, which are organic. The macrominerals are calcium, potassium, phosphorus, magnesium, sodium, chlorine, and sulfur. The microminerals are required in even smaller quantities and include elements such as iron, zinc, copper, fluoride, and iodine.

Vitamins can be fat soluble or water soluble, terms that describe how they interact with water molecules. Fat-soluble vitamins (A, D, E, and K) are absorbed by the small intestine with dietary fat and stay in our bodies longer, whereas the water-soluble vitamins (C and the B vitamins) are more quickly excreted through our sweat and urine.

Except for vitamin D, micronutrients cannot be synthesized by the body and must be consumed exogenously in the diet.

So how do you ensure that you're covering your micronutrient bases every day? Your best bet is to consume a variety of fruits and vegetables, plus meats, poultry, dairy, and grains on a regular basis.

MEAL TIMING AND MEAL FREQUENCY

I'm sure you've heard it all before: Eat smaller, more frequent meals to stoke the metabolic fire; always eat a nutritious breakfast, the most important meal of the day; and never, ever consume carbohydrate in the evening.

You'll see a lot of hullabaloo out there about what kind of feeding strategy is optimal to build a lean, svelte physique. You may be wondering whether you're doomed to nibbling on bite-sized meals for the remainder of your days. I certainly fell victim to this line of thinking several years ago. My meals consisted of 200- to 300-calorie morsels because that's what I was told I needed to eat if I wanted to continue burning body fat around the clock and prevent muscle degradation. No wonder I was hungry all the time!

The truth is, meal frequency doesn't matter much. From a body composition standpoint, the majority of recent studies fail to find a correlation between meal frequency and energy expenditure (Schoenfeld, Aragon, and Krieger 2015). The potential benefits of higher meal frequency may be negligible at best, and an irregular meal pattern may in fact have negative metabolic effects (Farshchi, Taylor, and Macdonald 2004).

What about nutrient timing? The idea of a postworkout anabolic window has become incredibly popular in recent years. The premise is that properly timing the ingestion of protein and carbohydrate around your workout can have a dramatic effect on body composition and muscle protein synthesis, perhaps more so than the overall daily intake of nutrients. This stance has recently been challenged by nutrition expert Alan Aragon and hypertrophy expert Brad Schoenfeld, who suggest that your total daily protein intake matters far more in the long haul than the nuances of nutrient timing (Aragon and Schoenfeld 2013).

At this point, then, meal frequency should be a matter of personal preference. Whether you want to consume eight smaller meals per day or three larger meals per day is entirely up to you.

SUPPLEMENTS

Fat-loss stimulants and water pills may seem enticing. After all, how nice would it be to veg on the couch watching sitcom after sitcom while three easy payments of $29.99 do the work of melting away your love handles? How silly of people to expend their effort in the gym and in the kitchen when all you have to do is fork over some cash to obtain your dream physique.

If it really were that easy, though, everyone would be walking around completely ripped. Yet as we can see, this is far from the case.

I recommend a generic multivitamin just to cover your nutrition bases. This suggestion is honestly not a big deal. Provided you have taken care of the more important tiers of the nutrition hierarchy, this idea should be only a blip on the radar. The absence of a daily multivitamin is unlikely to make or break you, but taking it can be beneficial, particularly if your calories are on the lower side or if your food choices do not vary much.

Fish oil is another supplement that I used to recommend to everyone, but it's not necessary for individuals who eat fatty fish on a regular basis (say two or three times a week). Additionally, research in recent years has found that contrary to what we once believed, fish oil actually provides little to no benefit for cardiovascular protection or body composition changes (Monaco, Mounsey, and Kottenstette 2013; Azin and Bikdeli 2014). Nevertheless, if you tend to avoid fatty fish, it probably wouldn't hurt to add in a few over-the-counter fish oil capsules to your diet throughout the week.

By and large, though, you should save your money rather than spend it on supplements. They are by far the least important aspect of nutrition, yet ironically, people tend to shell out hundreds of dollars on pills and powders they believe to be the latest magic cure. Focus on the bigger rocks of nutrition first—controlling total calorie intake, then macronutrient breakdown, then nutrient timing. If you do all that, investing in the right supplements may make the smallest of differences.

ADHERENCE

The year 2008 was when I discovered the wonderful and life-changing world of weightlifting. Along with that, I was introduced to the clean-eating craze. (For those of you unfamiliar with the concept, clean eating is about eating whole, unprocessed or minimally processed foods while eliminating "unclean" processed foods from your diet.) A lot of good came out of that. Whereas before I didn't quite understand that not all foods were created equal, I now was familiar with the importance of protein, and it finally clicked that eating right could help me both look and feel better. Within what seemed like a matter of days, I could look at any piece of food and immediately identify its primary macronutrients: Eggs contained protein and fat; ice cream contained carbohydrate and fat, and so on.

With this newfound knowledge, I changed my attitude toward nutrition. Rather than putting as little food on my plate as possible, I actively sought out meat, poultry, and eggs for protein; ate carbohydrate sources such as rice and potatoes, and sprinkled in fat-containing foods such as avocados and nuts.

At the same time, though, I also became incredibly confused. I was fortunate to have the World Wide Web at my fingertips (not to mention the advice of well-meaning friends and family), but the vast array of information seemed to contradict itself. One popular member of a fitness forum scoffed at anyone who dared to consume any added fat, whereas another encouraged people to down an entire handful of almonds a day. Self-proclaimed health experts warned not to eat past 6 p.m., and another budding fitness professional claimed that consuming most of your carbohydrate in the evening would turn your body into a fat-burning machine.

So I would try one approach and then another. I was easily distracted and unfocused, quickly changing course to follow the next shiny object that happened to pass my way.

Did any of the methods work? I'm sure they could have, had I stuck with anything for an appreciable length of time. I was too impatient, though, and I didn't like most of what I was doing. I was the ultimate program hopper, sticking to an approach for a maximum of two weeks before jumping ship to try something else.

I was so caught up in the hype of what was considered the ideal program that I didn't stop to consider how my preferences and lifestyle fit into the equation. In short, I overlooked one of the most important elements of nutrition: consistent adherence.

You can stay up all night trying to figure out what level of calorie intake will yield incredible fat-loss results for someone of your age, height, weight, body fat, and activity level. You can also split hairs over what specific exercises, rep ranges, and rest periods will maximize your muscle-gaining potential. This information matters, of course, and it's certainly something to consider. Equally important, however, is your adherence to your program.

A 2008 study compared the differences in dietary adherence and bodyweight change over a 12-month span between different popular diets (Alhassan et al., 2008). Participants were randomly assigned to one of four different diets: Atkins, Ornish, Zone, and LEARN. For the first two months of the dietary intervention, participants attended weekly meetings and read through their respective diet books, at the end of which time they were expected to have mastered their assigned diet. After this instructional period, they were told to continue to adhere to their diets for another 10 months.

As you might expect, macronutrient intake differed significantly between the four diet groups. The Atkins group had the lowest carbohydrate intake, while the Ornish group had the highest. Total energy intake, however, did not differ.

Researchers found that, regardless of the type of diet followed, those with higher adherence experienced greater weight loss compared with those with lower adherence.

Other studies support this finding. Westman and colleagues (2002) reported a significant relationship between dietary adherence and weight loss success in participants following a very-low carbohydrate diet for six months. As well, Dansinger and colleagues (2005) compared the Atkins, Ornish, Weight Watchers, and Zone Diets and noted that weight loss across was associated with self-reported dietary adherence but not with diet type.

The specific details of each study differ from one to the next, but the gist is the same: no matter how you choose to eat or what diet you're on, make sure that you can adhere to it consistently.

This is one of the most overlooked components of figuring out the right nutrition strategy for an individual. Yes, it's important to set the appropriate calorie intake tailored toward your goal, of course, but the nuances of day-to-day eating—the proportion of carbohydrates you consume relative to fats, meal frequency, meal timing, and so on—are what's going to determine how consistent you are.

Many people make the mistake of splitting hairs over what is considered to be the ideal or optimal diet out there without taking into consideration what's best for them.

The best way to ensure that your dietary adherence will remain high is to find a way of eating that you actually enjoy. If you look forward to your meals and like your diet, you're far more likely to keep sticking to it day after day. So while it may seem admirable and heroic to go on the latest crash diet, I'd actually argue that practicing consistent eating behaviors not just for one week or one month, but all year round is far more admirable. Like the way you eat! How about that for an original idea?

What this means is that being be on a subpar fitness program you can stick to consistently is better than adopting a program that, in theory, can yield quicker results but is difficult to adhere to. Crash diets are out; moderation is in!

ACTIONABLE ITEMS

- Rather than obsessing over nutrition minutiae such as whether a sweet potato has a better nutrition profile than a russet potato, focus on the big rocks of nutrition: calories first; followed by total macronutrient breakdown; then micronutrient content, meal timing and frequency; and finally supplements.
- Strive for approximately 1 gram of protein per pound (2.2 g per kg) of lean body mass per day, but don't get caught up in trying to get your intake exactly right.
- With carbohydrate and fat, start with a moderate intake and adjust according to your energy levels and personal preferences.
- Find the meal timing and frequency that works for you. Try consuming three larger meals per day with no snacks in between and pay attention to how you feel. If you don't like this schedule, you might want to experiment with six smaller meals per day or anywhere in between.
- Dietary adherence is just as important as the specifics of any nutrition program, so strive for high adherence regardless of what kind of regimen you're on. The program you'll stick to is one that you enjoy, so make sure you like the way you're eating.

CHAPTER 5

Living-Lean Guidelines

You'll notice that this section of the book is composed of guidelines, not rules. When it comes to nutrition, I'm leery of rules. First, what works for me may end up being disastrous for you and your lifestyle. Second, I believe that only a few rules apply to everyone. Ready for them? Here they are:

Stay hydrated.

Try to eat veggies.

Don't binge eat.

These rules don't require much elaboration, and for the most part, they are no-brainers. No one is going to argue that you're better off living in a constant state of dehydration. Vegetables are good for you—duh. And as far as binge eating, we'll dive into that later, but I think we can all agree that binging puts you on a slippery slope for continued harmful eating behaviors.

FIGURE OUT YOUR NUTRITION STRATEGY

Figuring out your nutrition strategy means finding a way of eating that best suits you. I liken this to dress shopping. You may find a cute maxi that the mannequin is wearing at your favorite boutique store. You eagerly try it on only to find that it extends 8 inches (20 cm) past your feet and hugs you in all the wrong places. It looked promising but simply didn't fit right. So you put it back, keep searching through the clothing racks until you find another dress that has potential, and then you try that on for size. You continue in this manner until you find a red slip dress with a thick belt that makes you feel sexy and confident. As a bonus, it's perfectly comfortable, and it looks as if it was made just for you. This is the one—you've found your dress!

Any nutrition strategy could potentially work if it meets the following criteria:

- Provides sufficient nutrients
- Works with your lifestyle
- Leaves you feeling your best, both physically and mentally

Whatever nutrition strategy you choose to adopt, the common denominator should be that you pay attention to your internal cues (how you're feeling, how the food tastes to you) rather than external cues (the size of your bowl, the time of day, your physical location). Indeed, research suggests that people with a higher body mass index (BMI) tend to rely on external cues to tell them when to stop eating (Sherwood et al. 2000).

This task is admittedly difficult. If eating right were easy, we wouldn't be battling an obesity problem. If it were a cakewalk, we wouldn't be struggling so much with maintaining weight loss.

I have friends who swear by Paleo, and others who are staunch advocates of intermittent fasting. That's all great. Rather than make blanket recommendations for everyone, I want you to stay open minded, experiment with various approaches, and find what works best for you.

Worry less about what you should be doing and start with what you can do and are willing to do consistently. If you're curious about any given nutrition strategy, I say try it out. Give it a solid two or three weeks. What's the worst that could happen? If you don't like the plan, go back to what you were doing before or find something else. No harm, no foul.

Recognize the difference between food noise and food voice. *Food noise* is allowing your eating decisions be dictated by distractions, peer pressure, and emotions; *food voice* is paying attention to both what you want and what you need and finding the intersection between the two. Food noise is reactive; food voice is proactive.

Don't be overwhelmed by what the media tell you is and is not good for your health. The flavor of the month used to be raspberry ketones, then it was gluten (or rather, lack thereof), and then it was juice cleanses. Who knows what the fad will be next month?

MEAL TIMING

You don't have to eat breakfast in the morning if you're not hungry and if you have no appetite. We have one camp that still likes to proclaim mightily that you must eat every two to three hours to stoke the metabolic fire, but that dictum has been proved not to be true (Taylor and Garrow 2001). Then at the opposite end, intermittent fasters are adamant about skipping breakfast (and intentionally restricting the feeding window overall) for extended lifespan, improved cardiovascular health, and enhanced brain function (Mattson and Wan 2005). The truth is that most studies looking at intermittent fasting have been conducted on either animals or people participating in Ramadan, and numerous design flaws have been pointed out in the existing research that makes bold claims.

The current verdict as it stands is this: The data are inconclusive at this time to make any hard and fast recommendations for the population one way or another. In addition, taking personal preference and individual response into account is important. Rather than sticking to dogma, find the approach that works best for you. See what I mean? Food voice.

When you do get hungry, rather than reach for the first edible item you see, take a moment to survey your options. Ideally, you will have done some planning and stocked your home (or your office or wherever you happen to be) with some healthy sources of food. After all, you're going to eat what you have access to and you're going to eat what you see (Wansink, Painter, and Lee 2006).

Ask yourself these questions:

- What do I want to eat?
- What will provide me with some valuable nutrients and keep me satiated?

Whatever that happens to be, eat that. Try to toss some protein in your meal if you find that it's lacking.

Table 5.1 gives examples of meals I might eat depending on my mood, energy level, and whether or not I'm exercising that day. Note that typically I have a higher carbohydrate intake when I have a workout planned for later and a higher fat intake for days off from the gym. This plan is largely by personal preference.

Table 5.1 Sample Meals

Exercising?	Sweet or savory?	Meal
Yes	Sweet	Protein pancakes with a light drizzling of syrup Shredded buffalo chicken breast Over-easy egg Black coffee with stevia
Yes	Sweet	Bagel with a thin layer of full-fat strawberry cream cheese Scrambled eggs with sliced deli meat Black coffee with stevia
Yes	Savory	Homemade skillet breakfast potatoes Scrambled eggs with spinach, mushrooms, onions, and cheddar cheese Black coffee with stevia
No	Sweet	Protein shake with chocolate whey protein, milk, peanut butter, walnuts, sweetened coconut flakes, and a handful of spinach Black coffee with stevia
No	Savory	Omelet with bacon, deli meat, spinach, and bell peppers, topped with sliced avocado Black coffee with stevia

Even if I do have something on the nutritionally devoid side (hello, pancake syrup!), I'll pair it with some quality protein. And if I do consume a lot of added sugars in one meal, I'll make sure to pull it in at my next meal and add extra veggies. I don't panic or stress out over any single thing I eat; nothing with nutrition is ever unfixable.

Checks and balances, y'all.

MEAL SIZE

Listening to your food voice does not mean shoveling down a bucketful of buttery popcorn every evening because your body was supposedly "crying out" for some salty goodness. You know when you're lying to yourself.

Again, take a beat. Do you find that you actually get hungrier when noshing down on a snack, or does the snack help to tide you over for a few hours until you sit down for your next real meal? I know that for me, snacks are mighty tasty, but they don't fill me up one bit. All they really do is give me something to do for three minutes and add unnecessary calories to my day.

If you find yourself constantly digging through the pantry for something to eat, perhaps it's a sign that the actual meals you consume aren't satiating enough for you. Maybe they didn't contain enough calories to fill you up, or perhaps the meals weren't quite what you were craving, so you were simply left wanting more.

One time a few years ago I had a hankering for a burrito all day. I spent the entire afternoon training my clients while salivating at thoughts of cheese, beans, rice, meat, and veggies all wrapped up in a giant flour tortilla. Mmmm. Nothing could have hit the spot better.

When I finally wrapped up work for the day, I walked over to Chipotle, only to find a long line that wrapped around the store. I decided it wasn't worth the wait and instead went home and dug through my pantry to find something to eat. Tuna straight out of the can. Frozen mixed berries with cottage cheese. Half a protein bar.

Those were all fine choices on their own. But every time I thought I was done eating, I'd find my mind wandering back to the burrito that I'd opted out of, and the craving never went away. So back I would go to the kitchen, sticking my nose in the cupboards, looking for something that would satisfy me.

By bedtime, I had consumed 500 to 800 extra calories beyond what I would have eaten had I simply honored my craving from the get-go—and I still wasn't feeling satisfied. It quickly became apparent to me that I should have just had the damn burrito! I'm sure something similar has happened to you, but I digress.

If you do decide that snacks help you, you have many options. In general, I recommend something nutrient dense, such as a piece of fruit and maybe a protein bar to pair with it. Or if you're hankering for something sweet, a square or two of chocolate may hit the spot for you alongside some Greek yogurt. (If you're wondering whether I'm intentionally recommending that you consume treats on occasion, you're not wrong. We'll dive more into that in the next section.) Here are some snack ideas:

- Protein bar with a glass of milk
- Apple with peanut butter
- Greek yogurt with mixed berries and a sprinkling of chocolate chips

- Tortilla chips portioned out into a small bowl with a side of salsa
- Carrot sticks with hummus
- One serving of gelato
- One brownie (the real kind!)
- Three cups of popcorn sprinkled with salt and butter

You'll notice that these snacks run the gamut from high fiber and nutrient dense to downright sugar laden. I'm not condoning a daily brownie; rather, I'm showing you that there's no right or wrong way to eat and that you never need to demonize any one food. When it comes down to it, you should probably consume the nutrient-devoid treats a little more sparingly, but having some every now and then is not going to make or break you.

MEAL COMPOSITION

Just about any particular way of eating has merit. The ketogenic diet, in which up to 75 percent of calories come from fat, 20 percent from protein, and just 5 percent from carbohydrate, is purported to result in greater net body-fat loss (Hall et al. 2015) and increased appetite suppression (Gibson et al. 2015). But other studies conducted under controlled, isocaloric conditions don't show any benefit of ketogenic diets over low-carbohydrate diets. On the opposite end of the spectrum, we have low-fat diets, in which only 15 to 30 percent of energy intake comes from fat (Lichtenstein, Van Horn, and Nutrition Committee 1998). Such diets have yielded greater weight-loss results over the short term (Lissner et al. 1987) but not over the long term (Karl and Roberts 2014). Low-carbohydrate diets derive less than 40 percent of energy from carbohydrate, and the findings pertaining to their effectiveness in inducing long-term weight loss have been mixed (Naude et al. 2014).

All these diets have one goal in common: to create a caloric deficit. I'll add that one of the most overlooked aspects of any nutrition program is your response to it: How do you feel eating this way? Do you enjoy it? Can you see yourself sticking to this program over the long haul?

Jumping on a nutrition bandwagon just because your buddies are doing the same would be listening to the food noise.

Remember that sustainability is the number one factor in nutrition success. If you can't stick to a diet, then the diet is not doing what it's supposed to do. Note that this goes not just for fat loss but for any other health goal.

I can't tell you which style of eating is going to work best for you. That would depend on your food preferences, tastes, and activity level. Drown out the food noise and pay attention to how you feel.

Is it scary that you have a choice in the matter? It shouldn't be. Having options should empower you to hone in on your hunger patterns, energy levels, and cravings. After all, the best nutrition strategy for you is one that you can follow, and the program you will follow over the long-term is one that you enjoy.

Your Questions Answered

Q: I was told that I shouldn't consume carbohydrate and fat in the same meal because doing so will stop the fat-burning process. Is this true?

A: This assertion is an urban myth that spread like wildfire about 10 years ago. People got scared into thinking that they could pair a protein (such as chicken breast) only with a carbohydrate (like white rice) or a fat (like avocado), but not both. Heaven forbid rice and avocado be eaten in the same meal! As you can imagine, this rule made consuming meals both impractical and unenjoyable. I'm sure that the idea of never being able to enjoy a juicy cheeseburger again in the name of fat loss seemed daunting for many. And cheese and crackers? Apple with peanut butter? Forget about it! Fortunately, we now know that mixed meals are perfectly fine. Remember the hierarchy of nutrition: As long as you keep overall calories in check, you can lose weight!

DON'T SETTLE; YOU HAVE THE RIGHT TO BE PICKY

When it comes to food, don't settle for mediocre. I'm not talking about buying only the most expensive gourmet organic foods that have been sprinkled with gold dust and blessed by a genie. You don't have to start grocery shopping exclusively at your local health food store. Taking that approach is all fine and well, and if that's your jam, then more power to you. I'm referring more to eating what you really want rather than going for a second-rate version that may ostensibly save you some calories but not satisfy you.

I'd much rather have a real, full-sugar, full-fat brownie with a scoop of slow-churned vanilla ice cream on top than a sugar-free "healthified" block of chalk with some half-calorie bogus ice treat. But that's just me. You know yourself best, of course. If you truly love some low-calorie concoction, then have at it.

The point is, whenever possible, you should opt for foods that satiate you. You will get more from your calorie expenditure, and you probably won't consume more than you need.

In a perfect world, you would always have access to exactly what you want to eat, but that's neither reasonable nor practical. What happens if you find yourself at a party? What happens if you're a guest at grandma's house, or if you go camping for a week with a group of friends? Life happens—now what?

Make portion control your friend. You can take this practice with you and use it anywhere, anytime, independent of what you're eating or whose company you're in. With portion control in your back pocket, you never have to worry about traveling or being away from the comfort of your kitchen.

Again, be picky. Load up on protein and vegetables whenever possible, and when it comes to the more calorically dense options, scale back on how much you put on your plate. Just because an apple pie is sitting in front of you, you are not obligated—by any means!—to consume the entire dessert.

Let's walk through an example scenario. Say I'm at a Sunday afternoon potluck, and I'm staring at a vast array of snack and food options—chips and guacamole, beans and rice, beef, chicken, and carnitas, an assortment of salsas and fajita veggies. At the end of the table is a plate of homemade brownies and chocolate chip cookies. It all looks delicious, and I'm starting to feel ravenous.

The default course of action for most people might be to grab the largest plate available and start loading up on anything and everything that looks delicious. A mound of guacamole here, some cheesy beans there, maybe a side of some beef. The more food options, the better! You're already planning to go back for seconds in about 10 minutes, and then later, to stuff as many brownies as you can into your mouth. You know you're going to eat yourself sick—you just know it!—because this is what always happens, without fail, at any buffet-style event you attend.

But this isn't what I would do. We're learning to be smart with our eating, remember?

Not surprisingly, researchers have discovered that folks with a lower BMI take more time to survey their options, leave more food on their plate, and chew more per bite of food when at a buffet compared with those with a higher BMI (Wansink and Payne 2008). This finding makes sense if you think about. By taking a few moments to take inventory of what's available to eat, you're essentially deciding what's worth the calories and what will satiate you the most. Then you end up consuming fewer calories than the average Joe, who might go into a buffet with the mindset that he has to eat his money's worth of food (when ironically, the health costs that he will have to pay in the long run if he keeps up these types of eating behaviors will greatly outweigh the price of an isolated meal). We can extrapolate from these study findings and say that people who are more overweight and obese practice the same health behaviors outside the buffet setting, thus partially accounting for their higher body weight.

Furthermore, the more food variety you have available, the more calories you are likely to consume (Rolls et al. 1981a). A study of 36 female nurses found that when presented with sandwiches containing one type of filling versus those that contained four types of fillings, the participants ate significantly less under the first condition. In another experiment, offering three flavors of yogurt as opposed to just one led to an average of 23 percent higher consumption.

Variety may not be the spice of life, after all, at least when it comes to making healthful choices. The cause may be that sensory satiety is food specific (Rolls et al. 1981b), meaning that the more you eat a food, the less pleasant it tastes, while the pleasantness of foods not consumed remain intact. (This can help explain why, after stuffing yourself silly at Thanksgiving dinner, you still somehow have an appetite for grandma's apple pie.) Thus, we can surmise that because buffets offer a seemingly endless selection of food and drink options and because satiety is specific to a given food, dining at these food havens can be a perfect storm for a calorie explosion.

The next time you're at a buffet, look around. You'll notice that, in general, the leaner people tend to have less on their plates, not to mention more vegetables and protein.

Circling back to the afternoon potluck, it's reasonable to assume that the chips and guacamole will taste scrumptious (can you say carbohydrate and fat?), and, of course, the brownies and cookies will surely delight anyone with the slightest sweet tooth. If I were to listen to the food noise, I'd take part in a one-person race to see how much food I could inhale in a 20-minute window. But my food voice is speaking up, loud and clear.

I want to have my cake and eat it, too. The good news is that doing so is entirely possible, both literally and figuratively. I just have to apply the checks-and-balances approach.

First, I have to make a judgment call. Of all the treats available, what sounds best to me? The brownies and chips are calling my name. That's fine, but I'll need to balance those foods with something healthier first. So I'll grab a plate and load up with the fajita veggies and a hefty serving of meat before adding a small handful of chips, a spoonful of guacamole, and one slice of brownie. This meal will give me enough of what I want (sugar! grease!) while ensuring that I get what I need.

Although you may not always be able to control what you eat, you can always control how much you eat.

This suggestion takes me to my next topic of discussion: clean-your-plate syndrome. This ailment, which I have previously been guilty of, is characterized by a compulsion to finish all the morsels on your plate, regardless of how you're feeling or how the food tastes. The causes of this behavior are numerous, including cultural factors, an aversion to food wasting, and plain old habit. But you're not doing yourself any favors by wiping your plate clean all the time no matter what. You're ignoring your food voice and instead relying on external cues to dictate your eating behaviors, which, as we know, can lead to some lousy habits.

If you're too full to finish what's on your plate, stop eating. Ask for a to-go box and save the rest for later. Chances are, if you're reading this, you're not living in a food-impoverished state. There's plenty of food to go around—in fact, there's an overabundance of food. You're not saving starving children in Africa by eating all your food, contrary to what your grandmother may have told you as a child.

Instead, let's get comfortable with a new way of thinking about portion sizes. You're done eating when one of two things happens:

1. You're feeling reasonably full.
2. The food no longer tastes amazing.

You owe yourself at least that much. You don't have to become a food snob; you can simply be judicious about what and how much you eat. The best thing you can do for yourself and others is to model healthy eating behaviors that others will see and eventually emulate.

MAKE MINDLESS EATING WORK IN YOUR FAVOR

You're at your 20-year high school reunion, and you're shocked to find that athletic jock Trevor isn't looking so athletic anymore. He has a hefty tire around his waist. You ask him how he's been doing, and he points at his gut and proclaims, "I don't even know how this happened!"

He's not the only one. I'm sure you know many people—and perhaps you're even one of them—who slowly pile on the body fat year after year and don't seem to realize it's happening until 30 pounds (15 kg) later. This phenomenon is common, and many people who gain weight in this way don't recall changing anything about their eating or exercise patterns (Sherwood et al. 2000). The extra eating was mindless, and the weight gain that happened went largely unnoticed.

The *mindless margin* describes the caloric range at which you are unable to detect the difference in nutrition intake. This amount is typically around 200 to 300 calories for most people. For example, if your usual intake is around 1,800 calories, you may not feel any different whether you consume 1,600 or 2,000 calories. If you were to ingest 1,000 calories, however, your stomach would probably be growling and you might feel lethargic. And with 3,000 calories, the food may sit a little heavier in your stomach. The mindless margin is that grey area where you feel just fine and don't notice small fluctuations.

This place can be dangerous, especially if we are consistently consuming a hundred extra calories more per day than we need. Over time, that can add up to unwanted flab padding our waistlines. The good news, however, is that we can flip that around. Instead of mindlessly eating more, we can rearrange our environment, mindlessly eat less, and make better food decisions overall. We can make mindless eating work in our favor.

The average person makes approximately 200 food decisions per day (Wansink and Sobal 2007). Do you catch yourself chowing down on the last handful of fries off your kid's plate? Munching through the stale pizza crust even when you're stuffed to the brim?

My good friend Karey and I once went to watch Adam Sandler and his crew put on a comedy show at the local convention center. She and I had just finished a big sushi dinner complete with appetizers, edamame, and sushi rolls. After making our way to the venue for the show, we ordered a large bucket of popcorn to share—it was an exciting night for both of us, after all. And then, within an hour of sitting down for the performance, we had cleaned out the entire bucket together.

We weren't even hungry. We had just eaten and were stuffed! Yet because we had food in front of us, we kept reaching for more. We mindlessly reached for more of the stale popcorn simply because it was there and within arms' reach. Neither of us realized how much we'd ingested until the bucket was empty. Because of the distraction of the show and the people around us, we ate until we couldn't anymore.

This example is the epitome of mindless eating. If food is in front of us, we're taught that our task is unfinished (Wansink 2004).

Much of our food decisions are mindless, and we don't even realize it. What's more, we are heavily influenced by what is around us, not exclusively by our hunger. The food available, the people we're with, the day it is, and the emotions we're feeling all play a role in deciding what and how much we eat.

Additionally, we're not very good at recalling how much we've eaten. And unless we have a visual reminder in front of us, we'll typically continue to eat the food that's available until it's gone (Wansink and Payne 2007). That basket of bread at the restaurant can be dangerous, and giant tubs of popcorn can get us into trouble.

But trying to be mindful of our surroundings all the time is a daunting task and a tiresome endeavor at best. Here's a story of how you can shape your environment in your favor so that you change your behavior by default.

In a six-month study in 2012, Thorndike and colleagues (2012) hypothesized that reorganizing how food was displayed in a hospital cafeteria would modify people's eating behavior. More specifically, they employed a *choice architecture* intervention, a term used to refer to the presentation of choice options. Perhaps the most interesting aspect of this study was phase 2, during which water bottles were moved from just two refrigerators located at an inconvenient location in the cafeteria to every refrigerator at eye level and in baskets near food stations. This simple change in presentation increased water sales by 25.8 percent, and soda sales dropped by 11.4 percent.

You see? Mindless.

This approach is clever because you're not relying on willpower and on exerting self-control, and you often won't realize that you're acting any differently. In addition, this idea takes advantage of the fact that habits rely on contextual cues (such as physical location) and that habits are not that strongly correlated with current goals (Neal et al. 2012). In other words, simply wanting to do something differently doesn't ensure that the right behaviors will occur on their own; interventions must be implemented to aid behavior change.

The ultimate goal when it comes to modifying your environment should be to make the target behavior the easier thing to do, not the harder one. The 2012 Thorndike study was effective because after the researchers redesigned the drink placement, reaching for a water bottle rather than a can of soda was the easier choice and required less work. Stanley Schachter found in a 1971 study that the more of a hassle it is to eat a given food, the less of it we'll consume (Schachter 1971). This outcome goes for both unhealthy foods and the nutrient-dense ones.

We thrive on convenience, and we're usually not willing to go out of our way to obtain something we want if we decide it's too much work. Something as seemingly miniscule as leaving the lid closed on an ice cream cart will mean that people will opt for a scoop half as often (Wansink and Painter 2005).

We can use this knowledge in our favor and make it more of a pain to eat junk food and to overeat. You can shape your environment for the better in an infinite number of ways. Here are some changes you can implement to modify your nutrition:

- Replace the candy jar on your desk with a bowl of fruit.
- Always keep fresh, ready-to-eat produce (e.g., carrot sticks, cherry tomatoes) in your fridge.
- Keep your fridge stocked with potatoes, rice, and protein cooked in bulk.
- Place the junk food (e.g., animal crackers, sugary cereal) high up in the pantry and the healthier choices (e.g., protein bars, old-fashioned oats) at eye level.
- Move full-sugar sodas to inconvenient, hard-to-get-to locations. Or better yet, remove them from your home altogether.
- Replace clear jars of treats with colored jars so that you can't readily see what's inside.
- Don't keep any indulgences in your home. Instead, save them for special occasions when you're out with your friends.
- Replace your giant plates with smaller dishes.
- Portion out your snacks onto a separate bowl or plate before consumption.

Willpower, not even once.

I want to hammer home this point because for whatever reason, common knowledge seems to be that we must rely on self-control to change our behavior. Although self-control certainly has its merits, those who attempt to rely solely on willpower tend to be unsuccessful in reaching and maintaining their fitness goals.

The term that scientists use is *ego depletion*, which is the idea that willpower draws from a limited resource pool and becomes drained with every act of impulse control, behavior inhibition, and decision making. (Note that recent research [Hagger and Chatzisarantis 2016] seems to indicate that willpower is in fact not limited, as found in the *Ego Depletion Registered Replication Report*. It's still too soon to come to any absolute conclusions. Nevertheless, what holds true for many is that exerting self-control absolutely *feels* fatiguing.) Baumeister and fellow researchers (1998) found through a number of studies that seemingly unrelated tasks of self-control (resisting chocolate and working on a difficult puzzle) depleted the same, not a different, source of willpower.

If you've ever wondered why you suddenly become far crankier when you're on a diet, this theory would explain it. Even the act of resisting a plate of cookies sitting in front of you is a form of impulse control, and yes, that act will drain your willpower!

Do you see how, when you have many responsibilities in your life, your willpower can become rapidly depleted? And do you see how this could eventually lead you to cave and do the very thing you've been actively trying to avoid? The more you rely on self-control to reach your goal, the more likely it is that you will eventually succumb.

I understand that we all like heroics, and you may want to brag that you're embarking on the latest extreme diet. Yet the United States spends more money than any other nation in the world on the diet and fat-loss industry—to the tune of several billion dollars—while also leading the world in obesity rates. Something seems a little off, if you ask me.

By modifying your behavior in a mindless, painless, habit-based manner, you gradually change your lifestyle to fall in love with your goal. Ultimately, this is the strategy that lasts.

AUTOMATE YOUR EATING

Back when I was in college, I would drive down the coast of California for spring break and stay at my aunt's home in the suburbs of Los Angeles for the week. For four years straight, I'd be coming off a grueling few days of finals. I was tired, drained, and aching for some rest.

I loved staying at my aunt's. The problem was that every time I'd visit, I'd find myself quietly digging through the kitchen pantry well past midnight, scooping spoonfuls of peanut butter into my mouth, scarfing down handfuls of cereal, and picking at leftovers. Why? Well, simply because that's what I'd always done at her house since my high school days.

This behavior is called an *eating script*, a specific automatic pattern of behavior related to food that we follow out of habit. Rhyme or reason doesn't always explain these eating scripts, and they often arise when we frequently encounter a given food situation. Here are some other examples of eating scripts:

- You smear the whole tab of butter onto your bread roll whenever you're at a restaurant and continue eating the rolls until your main meal arrives.
- You eat a bucket of buttery popcorn every time you watch a movie.
- You match your buddy drink for drink at the local bar on the weekend.
- You slurp on a vanilla milkshake as you weave in and out of traffic on your way home from work.
- You order dessert whenever you go out to eat with your significant other.

These behaviors certainly count as automated eating, but this type of behavior pattern will not serve us well in the long run. We can easily sabotage our efforts to get healthy if we continue with these mindless eating patterns.

One surprising finding by John de Castro (2000) was that eating with one other person increased food consumption by 35 percent; when eating with six or more people, you might eat up to 96 percent more than usual. Shocking, right? This outcome speaks volumes about the power of social norms. We tend to match the pace of our eating with that of those of around us, and we do the same with the quantity of our food intake (Herman, Roth, and Polivy 2003).

We rely on automated eating in a number of other ways to tell us what and how much to eat. The simple act of thinking that it's time for your meal can get you to eat, even if you're not hungry—and this behavior is especially prevalent among those who are overweight. Conversely, people who weigh less tend to rely more on an internal clock to determine when to eat (Weingarten 1984). We also eat more when we're distracted by watching television or reading the newspaper because we're not paying attention to the signals that tell us when to stop eating (Bellisle and Dalix 2001).

One of the biggest misconceptions surrounding diets and fat loss in general is that you must rely on willpower to white-knuckle your way to shimmying into those skinny jeans you've been eyeing. But we can't keep that up for long, and we're setting ourselves up for failure if we believe that weight loss is really all about self-control.

If we make hundreds of food-related decisions per day, coupled with the fact that willpower feels fatiguing (Gailliot et al. 2007), we may eventually run out of the mental fortitude needed to resist a pile of warm chocolate chip cookies.

I used to believe that the folks who were able to stay lean and maintain their body weight year round simply had more willpower than the rest of us. I envied them so! What I didn't understand was that it wasn't that they had more self-control; instead, they relied *less* on willpower to execute their daily health behaviors. How did they do that? Through habits, of course, by mindlessly eating better!

Over time, behaviors can become automatic by constant repetition (Ouellette and Wood 1998). In other words, you get good at what you practice. What we need to master, then, is how to adopt the right health behaviors in the first place. We'll cover that in the next chapter.

SLEEP WELL

The final living-lean guideline isn't specifically about nutrition, but it has a deep influence on the way you feel and the quality of the choices you make. Sleep is one of the most underrated determinants of health. A few extra quality hours of shut-eye can mean the difference between nailing that presentation at work and completely blanking in front of your coworkers.

One night of sleep deprivation can lead to decreased performance in simple, mundane tasks (Pilcher and Huffcutt 1996). Continued sleep deficits can negatively affect language skills, innovation, creativity, judgment, empathy, and tolerance for the new and unexpected, among a host of other measurements of performance (Thomas et al. 2000).

Insufficient sleep has been associated with higher rates of depression and mood disturbances (Rosen et al. 2006). This conclusion should come as no surprise. I'm sure you've experienced this firsthand when a night of iffy sleep has left you irritable, grumpy, and snappier than usual.

When you don't get sufficient, quality rest, you're not your usual self. You're not as happy and productive, and you're not nearly as pleasant to be around. You're a second-rate version of yourself. But how does lack of quality sleep affect you from a fat-loss standpoint?

From a behavioral perspective, sleep deprivation has been found to increase daily caloric intake (Bosy-Westphal 2008) and decrease energy expenditure (Benedict et al. 2011). Being tired can give you the munchies, in other words (Nedeltcheva et al. 2009), or make you not want to move as much. Going long enough without sufficient sleep can effectively stall fat-loss efforts and perhaps even lead to net weight gain.

Even if you're diligently adhering to your nutrition program and seemingly doing everything right, being in a sleep-deprived state can alter your physiology. In a study that compared people who logged 8.5 hours versus 5.5 hours of sleep during a caloric deficit (Nedeltcheva et al. 2009), the latter group lost more lean body mass, experienced altered substrate utilization, and felt hungrier.

How much sleep, then, is enough? Sleep needs are highly individual and vary drastically from one person to the next. Furthermore, it's not just sleep quantity that matters but also the quality. In fact, some researchers insist that quality is more important for overall well-being than the total number of hours of sleep (Pilcher, Ginter, and Sadowsky 1997).

Most people will do well with an average of seven to eight hours of rest per night. Some of you may find that you do better on more, and others on less. Moreover, consider *how* you've been sleeping. If you're a sensitive sleeper and are easily awakened by the slightest sounds and noise, you may want to invest in a noisemaker and some blackout curtains for your room. Making this one change recently in my sleeping habits has helped me rest far more peacefully and deeply.

When analyzing a fitness regimen, most are quick to slash calories or toss in more cardio, but they don't think about their sleep. Mindlessly moving more and eating less are not sustainable strategies, and opting to do these go-to strategies may be putting the cart before the horse. How *are* you sleeping?

The answer to your fat-loss frustrations may not be to do more in the gym. I suspect that many of you will benefit tremendously from simply making sleep a higher priority in your life.

We all have the same 24 hours per day. And although you understandably have some commitments that you can't do anything about, I bet that you have at least an hour or two of mucking around that you can cut out. Do you really need to scroll through social media before bed every night? Do you really have to spend your evening reading up the latest celebrity gossip?

Sleep is not for the weak; sleep is for the happy and lean.

ACTIONABLE ITEMS

- Listen to your food voice and be mindful of your internal cues rather than make poorly thought-out eating decisions based on food noise.
- Find a happy medium with your meals between what you want to eat and what will provide you with valuable nutrients and keep you satiated.
- If you know you're going to indulge later in the day or week, pull back when you can.
- Honor your cravings but be mindful of your portion sizes. A little can go a long way.
- Be picky with your treats and stop eating when you're either feeling reasonably full or when the food no longer tastes amazing.
- Mindlessly eat less by making the junk food in your immediate environment harder to reach, portion out your snacks into small bowls or plates, and keep your home stocked with healthy options.
- Strive for a minimum of seven to eight hours of quality shut-eye per night, both for your well-being and for fat-loss purposes.

CHAPTER 6

Embrace Moderation

I took my first foreign language class in sixth grade. I enrolled in Introductory Spanish, and as part of our homework, we had to choose a Spanish name for ourselves. On a whim, I chose Theresa. *Me llamo Theresa Lee y soy de Corea del Sur.* That was about the extent of my vocabulary on the first day.

As the weeks went on, we learned the Spanish alphabet and counted numbers. Eventually, we were able to string together basic sentences, however broken, and we communicated with one another with spurts of Spanish words combined with wild gesticulations.

The process was uncomfortable. I felt exposed, vulnerable, stripped of my powers. When it was my turn to speak, I froze, and every now and then I reverted to English because it was more familiar to me.

I took Spanish classes for five years, and by the end of that time, I was conversationally fluent in the language. I even spent the summer of 2006 in Madrid, wandering the streets and befriending locals on my own. What an experience that was! By that point, I was well versed in the language, and I could read the local newspaper and even follow along with the telenovelas with ease. I could call into a restaurant and place an order for takeout without a second thought, and I could engage comfortably in friendly banter with the grocery store owners.

To get to that point, though, I had to push through the discomfort of wading through unfamiliar territory for a long time. To grow, I had to fight the urge to retreat into my English language cocoon.

Think about the first time you tried to learn a new language or acquire any new skill. Developing moderation in your eating behaviors is going to feel like that at first. You may stumble in the beginning, and you'll likely be squirming in your seat. The impulse may initially be to cling to what you've known your entire adult life—perhaps restricting your intake and then inevitably going on a binge-eating episode. But what you've been doing up until now, however familiar, has not been working out too well for you. That's why you're here, isn't it?

The steps in this chapter may feel foreign to you, as if you're trying on a new pair of shoes. I encourage you to keep at it. Take things slowly, and if you're feeling overwhelmed, work on one small modification at a time. Eliciting lasting change is not an easy feat, and doing so requires an enormous amount of patience, consistency, and trust.

We're going to practice getting really skilled at moderation.

SWEET STUFF: ALLOW TREATS TO INCREASE ADHERENCE

Does the idea of cutting out your favorite foods forever and ever amen sound like an appealing strategy to you? Most people, when planning a diet, don't think about what they're going to do after the diet itself ends. They resort to drastic extremes—no bread! no added sugars!—thinking (mistakenly) that faster is better and failing to recognize that they will have to modify their daily health behaviors for life if they want to keep the weight off for good.

The norm for many yo-yo dieters is to be in one of two camps at any given time: They're either downing kale smoothies, crying over sad salads, and choking on dry chicken breasts, or they're inhaling entire pizzas, going on nightly frozen yogurt expeditions, and shoveling cookies into their faces as fast as possible. Because you only live once, right?

Remember, the best nutrition program for you is the one that allows you to keep deprivation to a minimum. Therefore, you need to incorporate some dietary relief into your program to keep the cravings at bay and to like how you're eating. Bringing back the idea of the mindless margin, the less you *feel* as if you're on a diet, the more successful you'll be in the long run.

I want you to practice saying this with me: There is no such thing as a good or bad food. There is no such thing as a good or bad food. There is no such thing as a good or bad food.

Now, let me clarify: Foods that are more nutrient dense should make up most of your diet, and foods that are less nutrient dense should make up a much smaller portion of your daily eating. We're not arguing that.

What I have a problem with is the demonizing of any one food, blaming one food for singlehandedly destroying your fat-loss efforts. Sure, painting food and drink in black and white is convenient and easy. I get that. It's easy, it's straightforward, and on the surface, it's a no-brainer!

But what happens when you deem a food off-limits? First, increased dietary restraint is highly correlated with binge-eating behavior (Marcus, Wing, and Lamparski 1985). In other words, the stricter you are with your food choices (and the shorter your approved food list is), the greater the probability is that you will fall off the wagon, so to speak, and blow your calorie intake plan out of the water. Likewise, rigid versus flexible dieting strategies have been found to be related to a higher BMI, disordered eating behavior, mood disturbances, and excessive concern with body size and shape (Stewart, Williamson, and White 2002).

And it's not just that. When you do indulge in "bad" behavior, you are then said to be "cheating" on your diet. What does cheating imply? You're engaging in taboo activity, which suggests sin, which begets guilt.

Furthermore, adopting the mentality that you are participating in a cheat meal—or eating a "bad" food—can be a slippery slope that takes you to larger, uncontrolled eating episodes. Oh shoot, you caved and had a donut that a coworker brought to work. Your diet is now obviously ruined by one 200-calorie treat. Logically, you could then go on an eating bender for the remainder of the day and inhale any "bad" food you're not allowed to eat until the sun goes down because there's no going back now. An extra unplanned 200 calories, after all, is pretty much the same as 2,000 extra calories—yep! (Please note the heavy sarcasm here.)

This behavior is the what-the-hell effect in action (McCann et al. 1992). The thinking goes along these lines: "Ah well, I've already broken the rule for the day; what the hell, might as well go all out!" This thinking is akin to finding that you have a flat tire and then stabbing a hole in your other three tires.

Black-and-white thinking may seem harmless in the short term but is disastrous in the long term. As you can imagine, the calories quickly accumulate, especially when you're reaching for the more palatable foods. For that reason, I'm a strong advocate of placing no food off limits and giving yourself permission to indulge. This approach can help you enjoy your diet, thus increasing overall adherence and leading to better results.

Although this suggestion may sound counterintuitive, I'd rather have you be consistently good enough and moderate with your nutrition every day of the year. Doing so will not only keep your body weight more stable but also improve your quality of life.

Note the difference between allowing yourself to eat treats versus becoming a straight-up glutton. Just because you can eat something doesn't mean you have to or that you should. Rather, you've shifted your mindset slightly: You have the freedom to eat what you want and the power to decide what's in your best interest.

If you decide to have a grilled chicken breast, a baked potato, and a cup of steamed broccoli for dinner, that's by choice. And if you follow that up with a small serving of frozen yogurt and a sprinkling of toppings, you have called the shots on your own. You're not following rigid rules or adhering to any kind of strict regimen; you're weighing your options and making the decisions that best serve you.

Some people like to call this *flexible dieting*. A number of misconceptions surround flexible dieting, so let's take a few moments to clear the air.

Myth: Flexible dieting is inherently unhealthy.

Reality: Flexible dieting *can* be unhealthy if you abuse it, but then technically it's no longer considered flexible dieting. It's not about seeing how much junk food you can fit into your day. By definition, flexible dieting primarily comprises whole, minimally processed foods and entails an overall mindfulness of macronutrient and micronutrient intake.

Myth: Flexible dieting consists of nothing but junk food.

Reality: Ah, social media can be extremely misleading sometimes, don't you think? Self-professed flexible dieters may proudly show off the treats that they can "get away" with—pictures of pizza, ice cream, and sugary cereal. You may conclude that these foods are all that a flexible dieter eats. In truth, however, added sugars make up approximately 10 to 20 percent of a person's food consumption, and this amount has been found to have no negative effect on overall health (Gibson 2007). We simply like to show those pictures because, let's face it, it's fun!

Myth: Flexible dieters have to count macronutrients.

Reality: To me, counting macronutrients means diligently weighing food with a food scale and tracking food and drink intake to regulate the consumption of a prescribed number of grams of protein, carbohydrate, and fat per day. And although many flexible-dieting people do choose to count macronutrients, particularly if they are preparing for a special event such as a photo shoot, competition, or other event where they want to look and feel their best, doing so is not a requirement. Being an intuitive eater is entirely possible on a flexible diet. The main difference is not so much in what your day-to-day eats look like but in the presence or absence of tallying up the macronutrient composition of your food. That's it. Actual food choices and portion sizes will be similar whether you choose to count macronutrients or eat intuitively.

Myth: You can't get lean by using flexible dieting.

Reality: I recently had a client reach out to me for help because she was in the middle of an argument with her husband about whether dairy was an impediment to losing body fat. She jokingly claimed that their marriage was on the line over this point of contention and that she was on the verge of losing her mind. To lose weight, you must be in a caloric deficit, however you choose to achieve that deficit (through curtailed caloric intake, increased exercise, or a combination of both); to gain weight, you must be in a caloric surplus (Schoeller 2009). More specifically, adequate protein intake and resistance training can help maintain, or even help increase, lean body mass while dieting down (Bryner et al. 1999; Norton and Wilson 2009; Phillips and Van Loon 2011). The only reason you should avoid a specific food is if you have an allergy or intolerance. Otherwise, overall calories matter first, followed by macronutrient breakdown, followed by micronutrients.

I don't want you getting your panties in a bunch over exactly what proportion of your diet any given treat takes up. Is it 13 or 22 percent? It doesn't matter, and splitting hairs like that is missing the forest for the trees. I also don't want you worrying about whether, say, a protein bar or a latte is considered acceptable. Again, that's not the point.

Your Questions Answered

Q: The idea of flexible dieting appeals to me, but I really don't care much for junk food, and I especially don't like donuts. How can I make this work for me?

A: Don't forget that the most critical component of flexible dieting is personal choice. If you don't like something, you don't have to eat it. The 20 percent upper limit for empty calories is just that—a limit. You are by no means required to consume junk food; it's simply available as an option. This subtle shift in mindset can help relieve any pressure regarding food restrictions and allow you to live guilt free and anxiety free.

I don't care much for labels, so if the thought of calling yourself a flexible dieter makes you squeamish, I understand. All the designation means is that you're someone who cares about your health and therefore eats well most of the time but also wants to be able to enjoy your life. That's you, right? OK. Then we agree here.

The 80–20 principle is a popular concept among flexible dieters that helps keep their diets in check. It posits that approximately 80 percent of your overall food choices should come from nutrient-dense foods, while the remaining 20 percent can come from sugary, greasy junk food. The whole purpose of this guideline is to emphasize that on most days, most of the time, your diet should consist primarily of whole, minimally processed foods. Think chicken breast, eggs, coconut oil, sweet potatoes, broccoli, kale, and all that fun stuff. You get the gist.

And the occasional scoop of gelato? That's not for your physiological benefit; that's for your sanity. Research has consistently shown that the more you place something off limits, the more you crave it (Polivy, Coleman, and Herman 2005). This is the opposite of what we want to have happen.

Do you really want to be the party pooper who refuses to go out with her friends out of fear of deviating from her incredibly strict meal plan? And when you go out, do you really want to ruin the fun for everyone and order nothing but a chicken salad, no croutons, no cheese, no cranberries, no fun? Oh, and hold the dressing.

Most diets include some degree of deprivation and denial. I don't know about you, but living a life of deprivation does not sound like a life I'd want to keep up for long, which is precisely why we have such trouble adhering to extreme diets.

Remember that the best diet for you is one that you.can adhere to consistently. You shouldn't feel as if you're on a diet (and you don't even have to be actively dieting). The best nutrition program in the world will be for naught if you can't stick to it, so let go of what is ideal and find a happy medium. Allowing some treats every now and then is a great way to enjoy the simple everyday pleasures and nip cravings in the bud before they spiral out of control.

Give yourself permission to have a life.

DOWNSIZE ME

Learning how to live a lean and healthy lifestyle isn't necessarily about consuming as few calories as possible. Although you do need to be in an energy deficit to lose weight, you still need to be eating enough to walk with a little pep in your step and hit your workouts with intensity.

In general, however, many of us struggle with eating more than we need. We don't want to be gluttons and ingest so much added sugar that we feel sluggish throughout the day, but we don't want to deprive ourselves to the point of suffering.

If you are truly craving something, then you should have some of it. If you don't care for it, then skip it. A little bit goes a long way, though, and you don't need to go hog wild with your portion sizes. If you buy a cookie the size of your head, do you really need to eat the entire thing in one sitting? Probably not.

Don't let the size of your plate or the size of the package determine how much you're going to eat. Food and drink portions here in the United States are ridiculous and have only grown over the years. Buying family-sized bags of crackers and shelling out an extra few cents to add a side of fries to your meal may be tempting, but the future cost you'll spend on diets will outweigh any short-term value you think you're getting now. You don't have to fall victim to this enticement.

As a general guideline, prioritize protein whenever you sit down to eat. Rather than whipping out a food scale or fretting over how many grams of protein is in your meat, try to pick a protein source approximately the size of your closed fist. I like this approach because it requires no math and no numbers, and it's proportional to your body.

Decide ahead of time how much you're going to eat. If in doubt, start small. Never eat straight out of the bag (unless it's a single-serving package). Instead, portion out your snack and put it on a plate. I recommend considering how active you plan to be that day. If you have a workout planned, then you may want a slightly bigger serving of carbohydrate. If you know you're going to be more sedentary, something like a side salad might make more sense.

The more calorically dense and nutrient devoid the food is, the smaller your portions should be. This guidance goes for both fatty cuts of meat and decadent desserts such as cheesecake. You may be surprised at how satisfying just a small sliver or square can be if you stay in the moment.

Whatever it is you're eating, you're done when the food doesn't taste as good anymore. If you continue eating beyond this point, you're simply adding calories to your day that you could easily do without. Slow down and pay attention to your food rather than scarf down your meal while distracted.

TAKE A BEAT

Are you hungry or just bored? Before poking your head in the kitchen pantry, be sure to determine your why. We often reach for food when we're not experiencing actual hunger. We may simply be thirsty or looking for something interesting to do to pass the time or trying to fill an emotional void.

If you find that you turn to comfort food when you're feeling sad, lonely, or stressed, replace eating with another activity. When you're looking for a short break from work, fixing yourself a cup of tea and calling a friend may provide you with what you're craving—companionship and camaraderie. If you're upset over a tiff with a family member, what you need is an empathetic ear, not a pint of gelato.

You may occasionally nosh on a snack for no other reason other than the fact that it's part of your eating script. But what if you were to consider how much it adds to your life, if at all? Downing that large buttered popcorn at the movie theater on Sunday may be a tradition you've upheld for years, but can you do away with it? That decision would save you over 1,000 greasy calories. If your reason for eating something is "just because," that's not enough of a reason. Cut it out.

Rather than impulsively grab whatever food is closest to you, check yourself. Determine whether you're feeling true, physical hunger or something different. Think about when your last meal was and what you ate. Think ahead to what you have going on for the rest of the day. If you know you have a celebratory dinner coming up in a few hours at the upmarket steakhouse that you go to only once a year, does the candy bar really make sense right now?

Weigh your options. Remember the study that compared the eating behaviors of lean people at a buffet with those of obese people? The former group took a few extra minutes to survey their options and then decide what they were going to put on their plates, whereas the latter dove right into the food and indiscriminately piled on anything that looked remotely tasty to them.

Take a beat.

Whatever you do, don't feel guilty. Life is too short to beat yourself up over a scoop of decadent ice cream. If you're going to enjoy a treat, make sure that it's truly worth the indulgence to you. And if you accidentally consume more than intended, no harm, no foul. Make your next meal better.

DRINK SMART

Back in 2008 my coach at the time instructed me, as he did all his clients, to aim for four liters of water a day. I was not told why; all I knew was that I was not to ask questions and to do as the plan dictated. Given the perfectionist that I was (and admittedly still am), I had a near-perfect streak of meeting my water goal for several months on end.

The problem was that I didn't know when to stop. I knew that water was important for my health, so I reasoned that the more water I ingested, the healthier and leaner I would be. As the weeks went by, my four liters of water a day gradually increased to five and then six until at one point, I was guzzling down eight liters every single day.

I'm sure you can imagine how this excessive water intake affected my life. Because I was a college student at the time, my days were filled with one class after the next. If I wasn't attending a lecture, I was probably either in the gym or studying. But with this outrageous water intake, I was getting up every 20 minutes to use the bathroom. Phew! This necessary activity not only cut into my work productivity but also was incredibly annoying, both for myself and for those around me. Talk about extreme.

Please don't make the same mistake I did. Staying hydrated is important, but at some point, enough is enough.

When it comes to drinking, I want to address two components. The first is your daily fluid intake, which is closely tied not only to your fat-loss efforts but also to your overall health. The second is alcohol, which, contrary to popular belief, can fit into a well-rounded diet as long as you take precautions.

WATER AND OTHER NONALCOHOLIC FLUIDS

For the purpose of simplicity, I'm going to lump all fluids except alcohol into one category. This group includes water, juice, milk, coffee, tea, diet soda, and so on. Despite the fact that coffee is purported to induce dehydration, the evidence suggests that this is not the case (Killer, Blannin, and Jeukendrup 2014).

Staying adequately hydrated from day to day is important not only for proper functioning of your organs but also for general well-being. With insufficient fluid intake, you can experience constipation, dry skin, headaches, and lethargy, among other symptoms. Losing as little as 2 percent of your body weight from water can lead to sizable drops in both aerobic performance and strength (Kraft et al. 2012).

How much fluid should you be consuming per day? As a rule, I recommend one liter plus an extra liter for every 100 pounds (45 kg) of body weight. If you weigh 120 pounds (54 kg), for example, then two liters or a little more should be your goal.

Of course, you have to consider individual hydration status. Depending on their physical activity level and sweat rate, two people of the same body weight may require drastically different quantities of fluid. Consider a person who is mostly sedentary throughout the day and lives in a cool, air-conditioned environment compared with a professional athlete who is training for four to six hours per day and lives in warmer conditions. Obviously, the two are going to have different hydration requirements.

Tailor your hydration needs to suit you as an individual. As long as you pee several times per day and your urine is mostly clear, you should be fine.

Now you may be appalled that I nonchalantly mentioned diet soda in passing. Many people are gravely concerned about the adverse health effects of nonnutritious sweetened beverages, and you may have heard that they can contribute to weight gain. I know I've certainly heard my share of remarks along the lines of, "You should know better than that!" and "Don't you know it causes cancer?" from well-meaning friends. But studies indicate that consumption of diet soda is not associated with higher body weight and in fact can aid in fat loss by curtailing calorie intake (Peters et al. 2015). No studies to date link consumption of diet soda with long-term health risks.

Your Questions Answered

Q: I've been told to avoid liquid calories at all costs. Does that mean I can never again enjoy a glass of orange juice if I want to be lean?

A: Remember the energy balance equation and the nutrition pyramid. When it comes to body weight, any fluctuations will be, in part, a function of how many total calories you're consuming relative to how much energy you are burning off. Orange juice and other liquid calories such as milk may not necessarily help you feel full, but if you enjoy consuming them, then I see no reason why you should hold back. Are the calories worth it to you? That's for you to decide. I enjoy a dash of half-and-half in my coffee every now and then, and I may drink a tall glass of milk to go along with the occasional cookie. My recommendation is to be mindful of the calories in question and consider that they can add up quickly.

ALCOHOL

Everyone knows a Beer Belly Bob. Whenever you see him, he always seems to have a beer in his hand and a gut to complete the look. With each passing year, his beer belly protrudes more, but one thing remains the same: He's always holding a beer.

This image alone may make you shudder at the thought of alcohol. You may be thinking that you'll have to give up your happy hour gin and tonic and your Sunday mimosas to get the body you want. Yes, alcohol does contain calories, and yes, too much alcohol can wreak havoc on your system, but you don't have to swear off it for good.

With Beer Belly Bob, the beer alone may not be causing his increasing waistline. Consuming enough alcohol can lower inhibitions and impair judgment and decision making (Li et al. 2009). Willpower, in other words, is shot, so all the work you've been putting in to behave in healthy ways goes out the window.

Alcohol consumption can lead to some, ah, questionable thinking, including a complete disregard for any nutrition program you are on. Suddenly, munching on the entire bowl of cheesy nachos doesn't sound like such a bad idea. And while you're at it, why not order a large pepperoni pizza all for yourself?

Lowered inhibitions because of alcohol coupled with the grub that suddenly seems irresistible is what can tip you over your calorie budget for the day. If you do this enough times, the excess energy can add up and become stored as unwanted body fat on your frame.

Alcohol by itself is not inherently fattening. A few beers a week, in other words, probably won't do any damage as long as you take into consideration its caloric intake. I am not condoning a steady diet of bourbon, but I also don't see anything wrong with the occasional glass of wine, particularly during social festivities.

Again, you must be consuming more calories than you need to gain weight. You can certainly enjoy a glass of Chardonnay and still shed body fat as long as you are in an energy deficit.

But we're not here to obsess about numbers. The last thing I want you to do is to interrogate the bartender about how many calories are in your martini when you should be catching up on the latest with your girlfriend. After all, who wants to be counting calories in the middle of social hour?

If you know you're going to be drinking later in the day, then come up with a system to ensure that you don't go overboard. The more specific you are about your boundaries, the better off you'll be. In addition, implement the nutrition checks and balances approach. Taking in calories from alcohol will necessarily increase your total energy input for the day unless you pull back somewhere else. I recommend reducing either your carbohydrate or fat intake, or perhaps both, in anticipation of the booze.

Here are some questions you should ask yourself before you take your first sip:

- What specific drinks am I going to have?
- How many drinks will I limit myself to? What is my stopping point?
- What food item can I omit from my day in anticipation of said drinks?

With alcohol, many of the same nutrition guidelines apply, but now you have to consider not only how many extra calories you'll be taking in but also how inebriated the alcohol will make you. Typically, the more calories that are in a drink, the smaller the quantity you should plan on having. In addition, if you're planning to pair alcohol with a food item, recognize that the calories can add up surprisingly quickly.

You know your own limits best. Be honest with how much alcohol you can tolerate. You can have it all—just not all at once.

Have I convinced you yet of the merits of moderation? Unfortunately, eating just one cookie isn't sexy or inherently exciting, but the payoff for your physique, your quality of life, and your overall well-being is priceless.

Getting good at moderation takes practice, so don't give up. Keep wading the waters of the grey area, even if you want to scurry back to your comfort zone. Mastering this skill is the key to living a thriving life that puts you in charge of your nutrition rather than the other way around.

In the coming chapters, we'll switch gears and discuss the last component of your fitness game: resistance training.

Let's plow ahead.

ACTIONABLE ITEMS

- Give yourself permission to indulge in treats every now and then to provide dietary relief and keep feelings of deprivation to a minimum.
- Cut calories that don't add to your quality of life and downsize portions whenever possible. Pour snacks onto a small plate or bowl, and when in doubt, start with a small serving. You can always add more to your plate if you're still hungry.
- Consume a protein source approximately the size of your closed fit every time you sit down to eat.
- The more calorically dense and nutrient devoid the food is, the smaller your portion should be. A little can go a long way.
- Take a beat before you eat something to decide whether you're truly hungry or just bored or stressed. Weigh your options and make sure that what you're about to eat is worth the indulgence.
- Stay hydrated with at least two liters of fluids a day.
- With alcohol, come up with a clear system to ensure that you don't go overboard. How many drinks will you have, and what kind? If you're going to imbibe, what aspect of your nutrition will you pull back on that day?

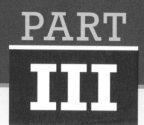

PART III

Lift

Resistance training is the fountain of youth. Lifting weights regularly has led both men and women to become healthier, stronger, and more confident across the board. Lifters, I've noticed, also tend to walk with a little extra pep in their step, and they look and move as though they are much younger than they truly are.

I've worked with thousands of women all around the world over the years. Admittedly, most of them come to me with the primary goal of shedding body fat and improving their body composition. I have yet to have anyone approach me and proclaim that all she wants to do is to be able to haul her mattress from the moving truck to her new home without any extra help.

I see nothing wrong with wanting to look better, to have a firmer, leaner physique with curves in all the right places. But along the way come a host of other benefits that help to improve your overall quality of life.

Part III is all about lifting. In chapter 7 I'll present an irrefutable case for why all women should embrace resistance training. You'll learn that resistance training is important not just for aesthetic purposes but also for health, function, and performance. In chapter 8 I'll walk you through the seven primary movement categories. You'll become well versed in how each exercise is classified, what muscles are worked, and how to execute proper form. Chapter 9 covers cardio and conditioning and includes glute circuits that both sculpt the derriere and create a good sweat. You may be surprised at how much you can do using just some resistance bands.

If you're jaded with your fitness program and you're ready for a lifestyle change that will have you looking and feeling your best, look no further than the weight room.

CHAPTER 7

Level Up With Resistance Training

Growing up, I was a relatively carefree kid. I stayed active through most of my elementary school years through swimming, running, and playing outdoor games with my friends. I'd play four square in the morning with my classmates while we waited for the school bus, I'd engage in a game of freeze tag during recess, and then I'd pedal my bike with my friends to the local park in the afternoon. Some days I'd even ride through the house on my scooter, gliding through the kitchen to slurp down some orange juice before rushing back outside to play. Hardly a day went by when I wouldn't be covered in sweat at some point. Physical movement was the norm, and exercise was genuinely fun.

I was a healthy child by all measures. Though petite framed, I was lively and energetic. I had a voracious appetite and ate what I wanted to my heart's content, which typically meant plenty of meat, rice, potatoes, and even vegetables. Occasionally, I'd enjoy a scoop of ice cream or a cookie, but never in unreasonable quantities. I ate when I was hungry and stopped when I was full.

Ah, how simple things used to be.

By the time I hit my teenage years, I was considerably more self-conscious and acutely aware of both how I looked and how others perceived me. Girls at this age become increasingly competitive with one another, and everything suddenly became a popularity contest. Being a fun person with a spunky personality wasn't enough anymore; now I had to wear the coolest shade of nail polish and rock a slim figure.

I was not a naturally thin girl, so this did not come easily for me. For the first time in my life, I started hesitating before reaching for the next chicken wing, and I made sure to eat less than my friends did. I noticed that the skinnier girls received more attention and were more popular, so I made sure to follow suit.

I started dieting at age 13. At first, it was relatively innocent—leaving a few extra bites of food on my plate and skipping my standard afternoon snack. But pretty soon, things started spiraling out of control. I ran for increasingly longer periods on the treadmill, and within months, I was forcing myself to work out for three hours a day through a combination of thousands (yes, thousands) of sit-ups, hundreds push-ups, and a mind-numbing amount of swimming, running, biking, and jumping rope.

I quickly grew to despise exercise. When I wasn't in the gym, I was thinking about it. And when I'd finally be done for the day, I'd collapse in relief. While my friends would meet up on the weekends to watch a movie and eat at restaurants, I'd duck away to spend my Friday evening quietly toiling away at the gym next to my home.

It wasn't that I wanted to live in misery; the truth was, that was all I knew. I thought that losing weight and being happy was all about eating as little as possible and exercising around the clock. I couldn't have been more wrong.

My dieting eventually morphed into anorexia, and my obsession with eating—or rather, with not eating—completely took over my life. I would go days without consuming a single calorie before being driven to the point of binge eating on several thousand calories in a one-hour sitting and then secretly throwing it all up. I lost my personality, I alienated myself from my friends, and my family watched in horror as I shrank before their very eyes. Once a healthy 5 feet, 2 inches (157 cm) and 100 pounds (45 kg), I found myself teetering at 80 pounds (36 kg) at my lowest point.

The kicker? I was the unhappiest I'd ever been.

Over the next several years, I continued to struggle with bulimia. My body weight slowly crept back up to a healthy level, but my lack of knowledge and proper guidance led me to continue to torture myself with exercise I despised, all in an ongoing pursuit of that slender physique. On the outside, I looked fit, but on the inside, I was still crying out for help.

It wasn't until January 2008 that I discovered that weightlifting was not only for men but for women as well. I happened upon the magazine aisle of the grocery store and stared, mesmerized, at a fitness model on the magazine cover. My jaw was practically on the floor. She looked at once feminine and athletic, lean and healthy.

So began my resistance-training journey. Seemingly overnight, I fell back in love with exercise and began to appreciate my body for what it was capable of doing. Rather than trying to become *less* of my body, I fell in love with lifting *more* and becoming stronger. I began to fuel my body with proper nutrients so that I could perform well in the gym, and I've never looked back.

Since then, I've tried just about every lifting trick in the book, from winging my workouts to body-part splits, from squatting several days a week to not squatting at all. I've competed in a bikini competition and won my pro card, and I've stepped on the platform as a powerlifter. Lifting has allowed me to learn to be happy with my current body while still striving for more. I spend far less time in the gym today—only a handful of hours per week—and I look the best I ever have.

Far more than that, however, I've found a way to make exercise not only enhance my life but also make me a more productive worker and improve my relationship with my friends and family. Resistance training saved my life.

For that reason, I believe that resistance training should be the mainstay of every woman's exercise regimen. Rather than defaulting to doing more cardio to get in shape and obsessing over burning calories, chasing strength in the key movement patterns will bring about incredible changes. If you want to build a stronger, leaner body, strength training is your answer. If you want to build confidence, lifting things up and putting them down will get the job done.

The main reasons that you should embrace resistance training are threefold: health, function and performance, and, of course, aesthetics.

HEALTH

A full discussion of the health benefits of regular resistance training could alone fill an entire book. Granted, the main reason that most people take to the gym in the first place is to look better—that is pretty much a given, and we'll dive into that at the end of this chapter. But resistance training has been shown to be critical in improving general health as well.

Not until 1990 did the American College of Sports Medicine (ACSM) recognize the importance of resistance training and recommend it as part of a comprehensive fitness program (American College of Sports Medicine 1990). Since then, resistance training has been growing in popularity among everyday folks who are realizing that lifting weights is not only for bodybuilders.

A consistent regimen of lifting weights can aid in increasing insulin sensitivity, basal metabolism, bone mineral density, high-density lipoprotein cholesterol, and triglycerides while decreasing visceral fat, low-density lipoprotein cholesterol, and triglycerides (Pratley et al. 1994; Winett and Carpinelli 2001). Moreover, resistance training is critical in the prevention and management of conditions such as low-back pain and discomfort from arthritis (Pollock and Vincent 1996).

Sedentary adults can lose from 3 to 8 percent of muscle mass per decade, which can decrease metabolism and increase body fat (Westcott 2012). Lifting regularly can be especially helpful to older adults, because it can help prevent or slow osteoporosis and sarcopenia (age-related muscle loss). Weightlifting also decreases susceptibility to falls and injuries. I find this last point particularly intriguing because I've met many older people who believe that they're simply too old to begin lifting when, in fact, they now have a greater need than ever to perform strength training. It's never too late to start.

All of this to say that resistance training is really good for your physical health. But it's more than that. Lifting is great for your mental health, too, and it can do a world of good for your overall happiness and well-being.

Amanda D. first came to me two years ago with the goal of shedding body fat and building muscle. She had tried seemingly every method under the sun and was at a loss as to why she wasn't seeing results. "In the beginning of my fitness journey, I avoided the weight area of the gym like the plague," she recalls. "I was intimidated because there were mostly men there."

But then she joined my online coaching community and became a part of a group of strong, empowering women. Although she had experience in weightlifting, for the first time she was following a structured training program, recording her workouts, and seeing her strength increase.

After a year of training correctly, her mind and body were completely transformed. Rather than trying to break down her body to fit an unrealistic mold because she was unhappy with herself, she changed her attitude to one of chasing strength and building herself up. "Knowing that I have deadlifted more than 200 pounds (90 kg) off the floor is one of the best feelings in the world," she writes. "The scale and food are no longer my enemy. I have become a more confident person, and I work toward encouraging other women to venture into the weight room and lift heavy things!"

Amanda is not alone in this outlook. Resistance training has pulled women out of depression, increased their confidence, and provided them with a newfound sense of self (Singh, Clements, and Fiatarone 1997). Women around the world have discovered through lifting weights that they are physically and mentally capable of much more than they ever thought possible.

The feeling of squatting your body weight for the first time or cranking out your first true chin-up—there's nothing quite like it.

For me personally, falling in love with weights helped take the focus off the circumference of my thighs and onto how much weight I could squat. Rather than obsessing over how I could become *less*, I wanted to lift *more*. Resistance training saved me from becoming swallowed whole by my eating disorders.

How refreshing.

After more than seven years of lifting recreationally, my coach and mentor Bret Contreras persuaded me to compete in a powerlifting meet in 2015. I had just wrapped up my bikini show and was looking for something else to focus on, so I agreed. I ended up deadlifting 226 pounds (102.5 kg) off the floor at 105 pounds (47.6 kg) of body weight. A year later, I pulled 248 pounds (112.5 kg), beating my previous personal record (PR) by 22 pounds (10 kg).

I never would have thought this possible in my wildest dreams. Up until about a month out from my meet, I had never been able to deadlift more than 175 pounds (79.4 kg). I may have simply lacked confidence, but mostly I simply never believed I could, so I never bothered trying. But with the encouragement of a trainer who knew what I was capable of, I was able to blast through that barrier and put over 50 pounds (22.7 kg) on my heaviest pull in a matter of weeks.

Just imagine how empowering it would be to achieve what you previously thought was impossible. Suddenly, you have a newfound sense of fearlessness that positively affects your life both in and out of the gym. You're no longer allowing yourself to become a victim of your circumstances; you're making your dreams a reality, getting out there, and busting through barriers. Through lifting, you learn to feel a sense of invincibility.

Life does not happen to you; you make it happen. You're in charge!

FUNCTION AND PERFORMANCE

My first internship out of college had me flying across the country to work at a baseball training facility near Boston, Massachusetts. Like most newly minted graduates, I had only the vaguest idea of what I wanted to do with my life (at the time, it was nothing more than, "I guess I like fitness"). Nevertheless, I was eager to dive into the real world.

I lived with two other interns that summer in a rickety house in Worcester. The only belongings I'd brought with me were what would fit into one large bag.

I worked as a strength and conditioning intern for three months before accepting my one full-time job offer at another facility, this time near West Hartford, Connecticut. I had two days to get settled into my new home before my 4:30 a.m. wake-up call to teach boot-camp classes.

On my last day in the Boston area, I was able to cram everything I owned into my Toyota RAV-4, including a portable air conditioner that I'd bought and a coffee table that the homeowner had given me. When I arrived in the town of Avon, I transported not only all my goods but also a brand new queen-size mattress up three flights of stairs into my apartment. The kicker was that I did this all on my own with no help from anyone.

Doing this was a huge deal to me. Just eight years earlier, I spent the summer before ninth grade taking summer classes at a boarding school, coincidentally not too far from Boston. I distinctly remember getting off the plane, scared out of my mind. I was halfway around the world from my family, and I was completely on my own for the first time in my life. As I stood by the conveyor belt in the baggage area of the airport, I nervously tapped my foot. I weighed 80 pounds (36 kg) soaking wet from hundreds of hours of cardio and months of depriving myself of sustenance. My backpack felt as if it were filled with rocks.

When my 50-pound (23 kg) bag came around, I feebly attempted to yank it onto the ground and had little success. I grew increasingly panicked as the bag moved along on the conveyor belt. My head grew hot; I could feel strangers watch me struggle in vain. Finally, a kind gentleman nearby, taking pity on this damsel in distress, lifted the bag up with one arm and set it in front me.

I'm worlds away from the girl I used to be, and I have no desire ever to go back there. I've since learned to pick up heavy things and put them down, over and over, until what once felt heavy has become light. Now when someone offers to help me carry heavy objects, I know I can do it on my own.

Do I need help with that? No thanks, I've got this.

Client Profile: Emily M., Age 58

It all started in late 2013 when my daughter shared an article with me from the *New York Post* titled "The New Pinup: Why Gentlemen Prefer Buff" (Amos 2013). My daughter had been weightlifting for about a year, and I'd never quite understood why. She encouraged me to read the article about how three fit models got in shape and got stronger at the same time.

We were intrigued by one of the trainers featured in the piece, Sohee Lee, and her philosophy to fitness. Before we knew it, both my daughter and I were devouring Sohee's blog posts and learning as much from her as we could. Even though I had been physically active for many years, this was my first time considering lifting heavy weights, and of course I was skeptical. Me, lifting those barbells? I thought I was more the 15-pound (7 kg) dumbbell type. But the more articles I read on Sohee's website, the more I thought, Why not? I can try it and see how it goes.

My daughter gave me one month of coaching with Sohee as a Christmas gift that year. She'd initially planned on signing me up for three months, but I insisted that one month was plenty. After all, I told her, I'm not the bodybuilder type.

Now almost three years later, I'm still training hard in the gym! Lifting weights has helped me build stronger and leaner muscles. Increasing strength through lifting has helped slow the process of normal bone loss and preserve the lean muscle that usually disappears during middle age. No medications needed!

I can change a 5-gallon (19 L) water bottle with ease. I can carry heavy boxes and help move furniture. I've gained confidence and can hang in the gym with the rest of the guys there. My husband is impressed with my strength and appreciative that I can help out.

This exercise routine has helped me stay healthy and maintain my physique. I'm in the best shape of my life at age 58—how many people can say that? I'm stronger and more energetic than before, all because of the power of resistance training.

I don't know anyone who ventures into the weight room with the sole purpose of eventually being able to haul their groceries into their home in one fell swoop, but it's certainly a nice side effect of gaining strength. Women from all walks of life report that resistance training has helped them complete everyday tasks that they used to struggle with.

They can move the couch on their own when vacuuming the house, haul bulky items to the post office, and perform many activities that they previously would have needed extra help with. That kind of independence is priceless.

AESTHETICS

This part is probably what most of you have been waiting for. There's nothing wrong with wanting to feel sexy in the skin you're in, my friend!

How many of you, at one point or another, have said that you simply want to "tone" your body? I know I certainly have. For many years, I fell for the false notion that logging more hours on the treadmill would give me the coveted look: flat abs, slim waist, firm arms and legs, and a perky little tushie to boot. It took me a long while to realize that I'd been searching for answers in all the wrong places.

When women say that they just want to tone, many don't realize that progressive resistance training will help accomplish the desired look. They seem to be under the impression that a heavy set of back squats will mean that you'll wake up the next morning with giant quadriceps muscles. I wish it were that easy!

Getting bulky from lifting is actually incredibly difficult for women, especially if they keep nutrition in check. The primary reason is that we women do not have

Client Profile: Jenny L., Age 36

I used to be a runner, but then I had kids. I went on walks and did light dumbbell circuits when I could. When my children grew to be toddlers, I decided to make time for myself again, so I returned to running. But then divorce happened. I found myself a single working mom with a home and a yard to take care of. I was pressed for time, and it was getting harder and harder to get a run in. Eventually, one thing led to another, and I stumbled into heavy lifting. And it changed my life.

I could always count on my "date" at the barbell. The bar was always waiting for me, pushing me, never mocking me. The bar was always there. It never disappointed. It was just me and the bar. I could push myself. I could concentrate on no one but myself. It made me stronger physically, and it made me a better friend and family member and, most important, a better mom to my kids.

When you lift heavy weight, you have to focus on the weight. If you don't, it will crush you. You must concentrate. It's just you and the bar. It's holy time.

I've since earned professional status as a bikini competitor, and I've also competed on the powerlifting platform. Lifting has changed my physique like running never could.

Resistance training has helped me find the best version of myself. I'm more than just a working, divorced mom. I'm a strong woman inside and out. I was made to do great things. I never miss a day at the bar because it never disappoints.

With lifting, there's nothing I can't do.

testosterone levels close to those of men to support appreciable muscle growth. In fact, the average male has 20 times as much testosterone as the average female does (Kraemer and Ratamess 2005).

Along these lines, I should mention the role that genetics plays in muscle building. Most women can go their whole lives lifting heavy weights and never come close to becoming bulky, but a small minority will indeed experience some pretty drastic muscle growth even with a moderate diet. A 2005 study by Hubal and colleagues involving 585 male and female subjects who followed a 12-week resistance-training protocol found that responses varied dramatically: Some people actually lost 2 percent of muscle cross-sectional areas, whereas others increased muscle cross-sectional areas by 59 percent. That range is considerable, wouldn't you say?

Without getting into the nitty-gritty science behind it, this discrepancy is largely caused by differences in satellite cell activation. Those who experience the most muscle and strength gains from lifting weights have more satellite cells surrounding their muscle fibers, which donate their nuclei into the muscles and signal them to grow. They also see enhanced muscle stem cell behavior and production of growth factors in response to training (Petrella et al. 2008).

Most people will fall into the middle of this genetic range, so chances are that you are in this category and can see mild muscle growth. This outcome is good. Contrary to what the media may have told you, having some muscle on your frame will give you curves in all the right places. Firm arms and sculpted glutes, anyone?

A few unfortunate people are poor responders, including me. I've been lifting since early 2008, and to this day I am told that I look like a naturally petite, slender woman. Most are shocked to learn that I can pull over twice my body weight off the floor.

If I spent my time bemoaning all the ways in which I'm genetically cursed, I would get myself nowhere fast. It's painstakingly difficult for me to build muscle and look as if I lift weights. I readily put on weight if I overindulge (and I swear that 80 percent of the extra body fat goes straight to my face), and my booty is inclined to be flat.

I can't change my genetics, and you can't change yours either. We don't get to go back in time and choose our parents. But we can do a lot through diet and exercise intervention to work on our weaknesses and maximize our potential.

After almost 10 years of lifting, I can proudly say that I've built a little bit of a booty for myself. Although my physique was always fairly straight up and down before, I can now wear a bikini and rock some curves, all because of years of intense, dedicated training in the gym. And although I will likely never be an elite-level bikini competitor, I'm happy that I've been able to transform my body. Year by year, I'll continue to make incremental improvements to my physique.

The approach may seem counterintuitive, but performing resistance training in a variety of repetition ranges—low, medium, and high—and striving to get stronger all across the board is what will help you attain that tight, lean, toned look you're going for.

And don't worry. As long as you follow a well-designed training program tailored to your specific goals, you don't have to be afraid of building gigantic traps or accidentally growing a thick, blocky waist. Exercise selection and program design will largely determine how your body responds to the resistance-training stimulus, and we'll learn more about all of that in the coming chapters.

Your Questions Answered

Q: How do I target a problem area? I've got extra fat on the back of my arms that I want to get rid of.

A: Ah, you're asking about spot reduction. This concept describes targeting specific areas of the body from which to lose body fat. For example, you may try to whittle away your love handles by performing hundreds of side bends. For arms, you might try to do a thousand triceps extensions. Studies show that spot reduction does not work (Ramírez-Campillo et al. 2013; Vispute et al. 2011) and that where you lose body fat depends largely on your genetics and gender (Pérusse et al. 1996; Kuk and Ross 2009).

But all is not lost. Although you can't control where you lose body fat, you can absolutely change the shape of your body by building muscle in specific areas, a phenomenon known as *spot enhancement*. Muscle, unlike body fat, is site specific (Wakahara et al. 2013). So if you want to give the illusion of having a smaller waist, you can build up your lats by performing lat pulldowns, chin-ups, and rows. And if you want to firm your arms, you can build muscle there through movements such as push-ups, triceps extensions, and triceps pushdowns. Decreasing overall body fat through dietary intervention (namely, eating in a caloric deficit while keeping protein intake high) can also help give you a slimmer, more athletic look.

Lifting weights regularly, however, does not give you license to overindulge in the kitchen and eat whatever you want. Please don't make this mistake, because consuming too many calories can mask all the hard work you've been putting into the gym.

When women bring up the concern that lifting makes people bulky, they're confusing correlation with causation. People often overestimate the number of calories they've burned during a workout and falsely believe that they've earned a giant plate of pasta or a greasy burger with a liberal side of cheese fries. This kind of behavior, repeated enough times, can put people in a caloric surplus. If you recall the basics of nutrition from chapter 4, when you consume more energy than you expend, you'll gain weight. This principle holds true even when you're doing resistance training.

Although lifting can indeed help build muscle, sloppy nutrition can lead to gaining body fat at the same time. And having both extra body fat and extra muscle can give the appearance of bulk.

By keeping your nutrition in check and chasing strength in the gym, chances are you'll never get too muscular for your own liking. The key is to find a balance between eating enough to continue getting stronger in the gym but not eating so much that your hard work is masked by unwanted flab.

Let's put the pink dumbbells away and start using the big-girl plates.

Client Profile: Jennifer B., Age 38

If you would have told me five years ago, "Jenni, at the age of 38, you'll be squatting 170 pounds (77 kg), benching 105 pounds (48 kg), and trap-bar deadlifting 215 pounds (98 kg)," I would have laughed at you. You see, I didn't exercise consistently until I was about to turn 35 years old. I grew up with relatively average genetics and was not an athlete, unless you consider dance and cheerleading a sport. I fainted after running 600 meters in third grade, and hence never got into cardio either. At 4 feet, 11 inches (150 cm) and stocky, my frame was suited only for activities like gymnastics, but I much preferred lying around on the couch.

My couch-potato days lasted throughout college and into my 30s. I dabbled with a trainer for six weeks at the age of 30, and from then until the age of 35 did next to nothing.

My mom, though—she was Superwoman. She worked a nine-to-five job, came home and cooked, and managed to work out six days a week in our living room following workout videos. I'd hear her huffing and puffing away, and honestly, it all sounded like too much for me. She would try to encourage me to work out with her—I went to the gym with her once and afterward couldn't walk for three days. She was energetic, in shape, ate well, and somehow managed to do it all. She even got certified as a personal trainer because she planned to retire at 65 and then train baby boomers like herself!

I lost my mom when I was 32, and her death devastated me. The thought of working out hit too close to home for me, and I continued to steer clear of the gym.

Finally, on the cusp of my 35th birthday, I knew something had to change. My digestion was terrible, I wasn't eating well, and I was tired all the time. I hired a personal trainer who worked out of a private studio. I signed up immediately for 30 sessions so that I was locked in.

She taught me the basics of the big three movements—squat, bench, and deadlift—and how to swing a kettlebell and perform accessory work. I realized pretty quickly, as did she, that despite my couch-potato tendencies, I had a natural muscular base and was actually pretty strong.

Each week, I'd get excited to go lift and reach new personal records. In late 2014 I wanted to take it to the next level and work out on my own, so I hired Sohee for guidance on training and nutrition programming.

I'm now a certified personal trainer and working toward getting my nutrition certification. I lift heavy three or four times per week, and I genuinely look forward to my time in the gym. It's my me-time; my time to de-stress and feel close to my mother. During my heavy lifts, I talk to her, I think of her, and I feel her with me. I know that if she were alive, we'd be doing the same program and comparing our weightlifting numbers.

The person I am today is a better person for having resistance training in my life. The benefits are numerous—my arms, abs, legs, and butt all look 10 times better than they did three years ago, not to mention I look 10 years younger than I am because my body is able to stay in shape and keep me youthful. My overall health is better—my digestion, cholesterol, and eating habits are improved. My mental health is stable. I am a happier, less stressed, more energetic Jenni than I was before. I feel as if I can handle anything that comes my way.

My only regret is that I didn't realize this sooner and enjoy resistance training with my mom when she was alive. That said, I am happy that I found my passion, and it happens to bring me closer to my mom.

ACTIONABLE ITEMS

- Lift weights regularly to improve health markers, prevent and mitigate chronic conditions, boost confidence, and perform better in your day-to-day life.
- Don't be afraid of getting bulky from resistance training. The toned look that many women covet requires having some muscle mass in the right places. As long as you keep your nutrition in check, you'll look leaner and more athletic.
- Train in all repetition ranges (low, medium, and high) and push your effort in the gym to optimize muscle growth and strength gains.

CHAPTER 8

Primary Strength Movements

In this chapter, I walk you through all the exercises you'll need to know to complete my training programs. I take you through the setup and execution and go over some important tips.

I've divided the exercises into seven movement categories. Study each movement carefully; eventually, they should become second nature to you.

Familiarizing yourself with proper form should be of paramount importance. Master form first before adding load. In this way, you'll not only work the proper muscles but also stay injury free.

SQUAT

The squat is a knee-dominant movement that involves deep flexion in the knees and hips. Exercises that fit in this category work the quadriceps and erector spinae to a high degree. Contrary to popular belief, however, squats are not necessarily the best for building the glutes.

The most popular lower-body exercises fall into this category, such as the back squat, goblet squat, and Bulgarian split squat.

In figure 8.1, note how the squat looks from the front and from the side. Note how the knees are shoved out, the chest stays up, and the back stays in a neutral position. These basic cues go along with all squat pattern movements.

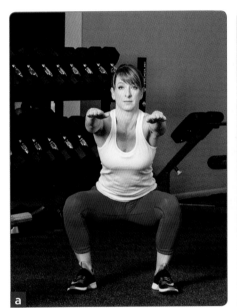 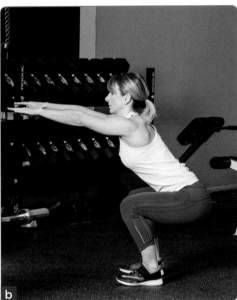

Figure 8.1 Squat: *(a)* front view; *(b)* side view.

Many people mistakenly believe that they're simply not cut out to be good squatters. After practicing the movement pattern with good form, however, they realize that this is not the case.

Beginners should start with the box squat and progress from there. When you can perform 20 bodyweight repetitions of the box squat with quality form, you're ready to add load and progress to other squat variations, such as the goblet squat and front squat.

BODYWEIGHT BOX SQUAT

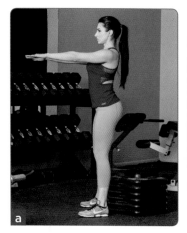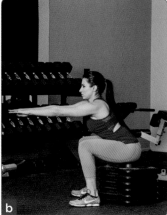

Figure 8.2   Bodyweight box squat: *(a)* starting position; *(b)* squat.

MUSCLES

Primary: quadriceps, gluteals, erector spinae

Secondary: hamstrings, adductors

MOVEMENT

1. Stand in front of a box squat box, plyo box, or weight bench 11 to 16 inches (28 to 41 cm) tall. Stand close to the box or straddle it slightly.
2. Position your feet slightly wider than shoulder-width apart and flare your feet out 30 to 45 degrees.
3. Sit back and lower yourself onto the box in a controlled manner while keeping your shins vertical and knees pushed out.
4. When you reach a seated position, pause briefly while keeping your low back arched.
5. Reverse the motion by pushing through your heels. Squeeze the glutes to lockout.

TIPS

- This movement is not how you will normally squat. It's a drill to teach you to use your hips more.
- The ideal foot stance will vary from one person to the next. Tinker with your foot position and find what feels best for you and allows you to perform the movement with proper form.
- Take your time sitting back onto the box and be careful not to plop. You should feel a good stretch in your hamstrings.
- Imagine that someone is standing behind you with a rope around your hips and pulling back.
- With deep box squats, in which the hip joint is lower than the knee joint, you won't be able to keep your shins vertical; the knees must come forward a little bit to achieve depth. This is not the case with parallel box squats, however, in which the hip joint is in line with the knee joint.

Variation 1: Dumbbell Goblet Box Squat

Hold a dumbbell vertically, resting it on your palms and pressing it up against your chest as you perform the box squat.

Variation 2: Barbell Box Squat

Brace a barbell against your upper back as you perform the box squat.

DUMBBELL GOBLET SQUAT

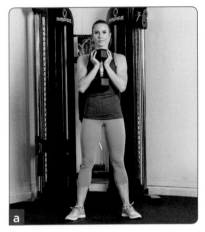 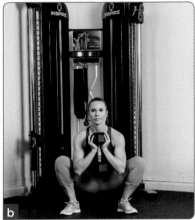

Figure 8.3 Dumbbell goblet squat: *(a)* starting position; *(b)* squat.

MUSCLES

Primary: quadriceps, gluteals, erector spinae

Secondary: hamstrings, adductors

MOVEMENT

1. Stand and hold a dumbbell against your chest, resting the dumbbell on your palms.
2. Position your feet slightly wider than shoulder-width apart and flare your feet out 30 to 45 degrees.
3. Take in a deep breath and drop your hips straight down in a controlled manner while pushing your knees out and staying as upright as possible. Your elbows should stay between your knees at all times.
4. Squat down until your hip crease is in line with your knee joint or lower.
5. Reverse the motion by pushing through your heels and breathe out during the ascent. Squeeze the glutes to lockout.

TIPS

- Some people like to use a wide stance with the goblet squat, which is fine, but I prefer a medium stance with the knees flared out.
- Keep your chest up throughout the entire range of motion.
- Actively push your knees out, especially as you come up out of the bottom of the squat.
- Point your elbows down, not out.

Variation 1: Knee-Banded Dumbbell Goblet Squat

Perform the dumbbell goblet squat with a miniband wrapped just below the knees.

Variation 2: Kettlebell Goblet Squat

Perform the traditional kettlebell goblet squat with the kettlebell held up against your chest by the handles.

Variation 3: Knee-Banded Kettlebell Goblet Squat

Perform the traditional kettlebell goblet squat with a miniband wrapped at or just below the knees (figure 8.4).

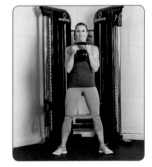

Figure 8.4 Knee-banded kettlebell goblet squat, starting position.

BARBELL FRONT SQUAT

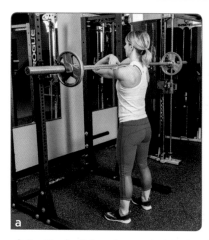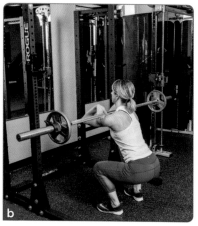

Figure 8.5 Barbell front squat: (*a*) starting position; (*b*) squat.

MUSCLES

Primary: quadriceps, gluteals, erector spinae

Secondary: hamstrings, adductors

MOVEMENT

1. Walk up to a barbell in a squat rack at approximately shoulder height. Unrack the barbell so that it hugs your neck. Take two or three controlled steps back away from the squat rack.
2. Position your feet slightly wider than shoulder-width apart and flare your feet out 30 to 45 degrees.
3. Take in a deep breath and drop straight down in a controlled manner while pushing your knees out and staying as upright as possible.
4. Squat down until your hip crease is in line with your knee joint or lower.
5. Reverse the motion by pushing through your heels and breathe out during the ascent. Squeeze the glutes to lockout.
6. After performing all repetitions, rerack the barbell by taking two or three controlled steps forward. Without turning your head, listen to the barbell tap the rack and then lower it onto the supports.

TIPS

- Rather than sit back, sit straight down and keep the torso as vertical as possible.
- A common mistake that lifters make is letting their elbows drop on the descent, which causes them to fall forward. Make an effort to shove the elbows up.
- You can use a clean grip, in which you hold onto the barbell with the ends of your index and middle fingers, or a cross grip, in which you cross your arms in front of you. You may find the latter variation more comfortable.
- You may find that wearing squat shoes or sliding weight plates under your heels is helpful in achieving proper depth and maintaining quality form.

BARBELL BACK SQUAT

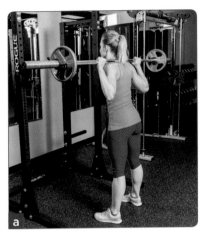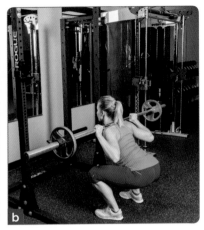

Figure 8.6 Barbell back squat: *(a)* starting position; *(b)* squat.

MUSCLES

Primary: quadriceps, gluteals, erector spinae

Secondary: hamstrings, adductors

MOVEMENT

1. Walk up to a barbell in a squat rack at approximately shoulder height.
2. Get under the barbell and unrack it so that it rests across your upper back.
3. Take two or three controlled steps back away from the rack.
4. Position your feet slightly wider than shoulder-width apart and flare your feet out 30 to 45 degrees.
5. Take in a deep breath and drop straight down in a controlled manner while pushing your knees out and staying as upright as possible.
6. Squat down until your hip crease is in line with your knee joint or lower.
7. Reverse the motion by pushing through your heels and exhale during the ascent. Squeeze the glutes to lockout.
8. After performing all repetitions, rerack the barbell by taking two or three controlled steps forward. Without turning your head, listen to the barbell tap the rack and then lower it onto the supports.

TIPS

- If your femurs are long relative to your total height or your hips are stronger relative to your quadriceps, you'll likely have more forward lean than the average lifter. Still, you should strive to maintain a relatively consistent torso angle through the duration of the movement.
- Most women prefer high-bar squats, in which the barbell sits on top of the trapezius muscles. But if they take the time to learn low-bar squats, in which the barbell sits approximately 3 inches (7.5 cm) lower on the rear deltoids, many learn to like this variation and can typically lift approximately 10 percent more weight. If you're prone to wrist pain during low-bar squats because of wrist hyperextension, you may find wrist wraps helpful.
- You may find that wearing squat shoes or sliding weight plates under your heels is helpful in achieving proper depth and maintaining quality form.

DUMBBELL SUMO SQUAT

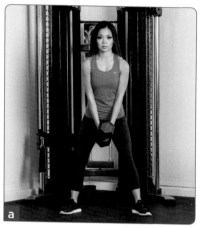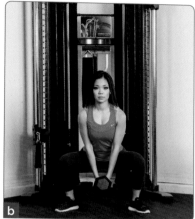

Figure 8.7 Dumbbell sumo squat: *(a)* starting position; *(b)* squat.

MUSCLES

Primary: quadriceps, gluteals, erector spinae

Secondary: hamstrings, adductors

MOVEMENT

1. Hold a dumbbell between your legs and grip the handle with both hands.
2. Position your feet in a wide sumo stance several inches (cm) outside shoulder width and flare your feet out 30 to 45 degrees.
3. Take in a deep breath and drop straight down in a controlled manner while pushing your knees out and staying as upright as possible.
4. Squat down until your hip crease is in line with your knee joint or lower.
5. Reverse the motion by pushing through your heels and breathe out during the ascent. Squeeze the glutes to lockout.

TIPS

- With this exercise, your torso should be much more upright and you should feel your quads working a lot more than they do in the back squat.
- Because you're going to be limited by your grip, you can increase the difficulty of this movement by adding a five-second pause at the bottom of each repetition.
- Keep the shins roughly vertical with this movement and ensure that your knees track over your toes.

BODYWEIGHT SPLIT SQUAT

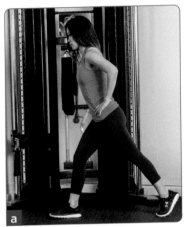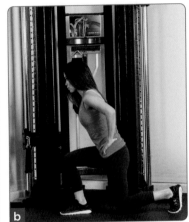

Figure 8.8 Bodyweight split squat: *(a)* starting position; *(b)* squat.

MUSCLES

Primary: quadriceps, gluteals

Secondary: hamstrings, adductors

MOVEMENT

1. Assume a staggered stance with your hands on your hips.
2. Drop the back knee toward the ground in a controlled manner, keeping the torso relatively upright.
3. Graze the ground with your back knee and reverse the motion, pushing through your front heel.
4. After completing the desired number of repetitions on one side, switch legs and repeat.

TIPS

- To target more of your quadriceps, stay more upright; to target more of your glutes, bend more at the hips.
- Think of keeping most of your load on your front leg.
- Besides adding load, you can increase the difficulty of this movement by performing it constant-tension style, using rapid speed, and not going to full lockout at the top of each repetition.

Variation 1: Dumbbell Split Squat

Perform the split squat while holding a dumbbell in both hands by your sides.

Variation 2: Barbell Split Squat

Perform the split squat while holding a barbell braced across your upper back.

BODYWEIGHT WALKING LUNGE

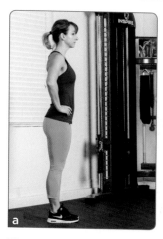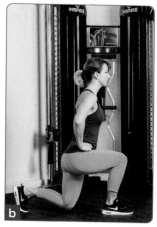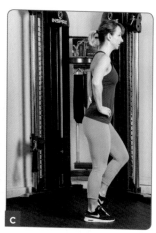

Figure 8.9 Bodyweight walking lunge: *(a)* starting position; *(b)* lunge; *(c)* step forward with other leg.

MUSCLES

Primary: quadriceps, gluteals

Secondary: hamstrings, adductors

MOVEMENT

1. Stand tall with your hands on your hips.
2. Take one step forward while simultaneously dropping the knee of the back leg toward the ground in a controlled manner, keeping the torso relatively upright.
3. Graze the ground with the knee of the back leg and then push off the toes of the back leg to step forward.
4. Repeat the movement with the opposite leg.

TIPS

- To target more of your quadriceps, take short strides; to target more of your adductors and gluteals, take longer strides.
- The back knee should be roughly in line with the front toe at the bottom of the movement.

Variation 1: Dumbbell Walking Lunge

Perform the walking lunge while holding a dumbbell in each hand by your sides.

Variation 2: Barbell Walking Lunge

Perform the walking lunge while holding a barbell braced across your upper back.

BODYWEIGHT REVERSE LUNGE

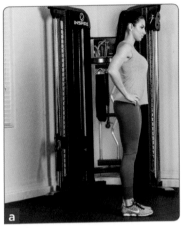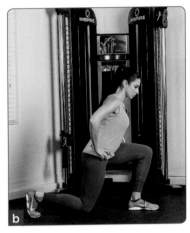

Figure 8.10 Bodyweight reverse lunge: (a) starting position; (b) lunge.

MUSCLES

Primary: quadriceps, gluteals

Secondary: hamstrings, adductors

MOVEMENT

1. Stand tall with your hands on your hips.
2. Step back while simultaneously dropping the knee of the back leg toward the ground in a controlled manner, keeping the torso relatively upright.
3. Graze the ground with the knee of the back leg and then push off the toes of the same leg to return to the starting position.
4. Repeat the movement with the opposite leg.

TIPS

- Don't let your hips shoot up or your depth diminish as you fatigue.
- Don't worry if you lose your balance on a few repetitions. This breakdown is common, and you should improve over time.
- You can perform all prescribed repetitions on one leg before switching sides to induce greater tension, or you can switch legs with every repetition.

Variation 1: Dumbbell Reverse Lunge

Perform the reverse lunge while holding a dumbbell in each hand by your sides.

Variation 2: Barbell Reverse Lunge

Perform the reverse lunge while holding a barbell braced across your upper back.

BODYWEIGHT DEFICIT REVERSE LUNGE

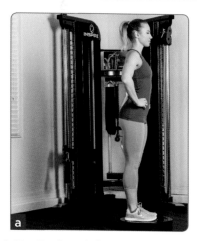 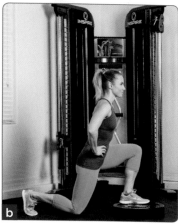

Figure 8.11 Bodyweight deficit reverse lunge: *(a)* starting position; *(b)* lunge.

MUSCLES

Primary: quadriceps, gluteals

Secondary: hamstrings, adductors

MOVEMENT

1. Stand on a platform 4 to 8 inches (10 to 20 cm) tall.
2. Step back while simultaneously dropping the knee of the back leg toward the ground in a controlled manner, keeping the torso relatively upright.
3. Graze the ground with the knee of the back leg and then push off the toes of the same leg to return to the starting position.
4. Repeat the movement with the opposite leg.

TIPS

- Relative to the regular reverse lunge, you can let your front knee travel forward more and stay more upright with the deficit reverse lunge.
- You can perform all prescribed repetitions on one leg before switching sides to induce greater tension, or you can switch legs with every repetition.
- The greater the height of the platform is, the more difficult the movement will be. If you choose to add weight, as in the variations, adjust your load accordingly.

Variation 1: Dumbbell Deficit Reverse Lunge

Perform the deficit reverse lunge while holding a dumbbell in each hand by your sides.

Variation 2: Barbell Deficit Reverse Lunge

Perform the reverse lunge while holding a barbell braced across your upper back.

BODYWEIGHT STEP-UP

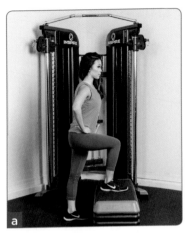 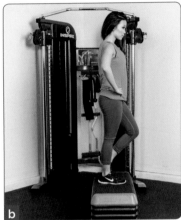

Figure 8.12 Bodyweight step-up: *(a)* starting position; *(b)* step-up.

MUSCLES

Primary: quadriceps, gluteals

Secondary: hamstrings, adductors

MOVEMENT

1. Stand facing a bench or a platform that is 10 to 20 inches (25 to 50 cm) tall.
2. Lift one leg and place the entire foot on the platform.
3. Push through the heel of the top leg and step up onto the platform, squeezing the glutes at lockout.
4. Without touching the foot of the trailing leg to the platform, reverse the motion in a controlled manner while keeping the foot of the front leg stationary.
5. After completing the desired number of repetitions on one side, switch legs and repeat.

TIPS

- To target more of your quadriceps, stay more upright; to target more of your glutes, bend more at the hips. If you're leaning forward more, don't let your hips shoot up.
- Ensure that your entire foot is on the platform; otherwise, you won't be able to push through the heel.
- Don't rely too much on momentum to step up.
- If you're new to the step-up exercise, start with a lower platform. You can use a higher step as you improve coordination and increase strength over time.

Variation: Dumbbell Step-Up

Perform the step-up while holding a dumbbell in each hand by your sides.

HIGH STEP-UP

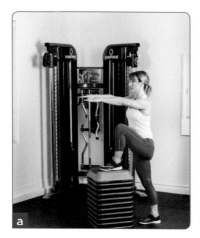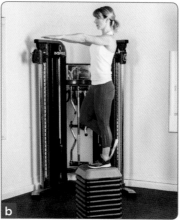

Figure 8.13 High step-up: *(a)* starting position; *(b)* step-up.

MUSCLES
Primary: quadriceps, gluteals

Secondary: hamstrings, adductors

MOVEMENT
1. Stand facing a bench or a platform that is 30 to 46 inches (75 to 115 cm) tall.
2. Lift one leg and place the entire foot on the platform.
3. Push through the heel of the top leg and step up onto the platform, squeezing the glutes at lockout.
4. Without touching the foot of the trailing leg to the platform, reverse the motion in a controlled manner while keeping the foot of the front leg stationary.
5. After completing the desired number of repetitions on one side, switch legs and repeat.

TIPS
- Ensure that your entire foot is on the platform; otherwise, you won't be able to push through the heel.
- Don't rely too much on momentum to step up.
- The bottom position of the high step-up mimics the back squat because the working leg is in the same position at the bottom of a deep squat. With that said, don't choose a platform height so high that your low back rounds.

Variation: Dumbbell High Step-Up
Perform the step-up while holding a dumbbell in each hand by your sides.

BODYWEIGHT BULGARIAN SPLIT SQUAT

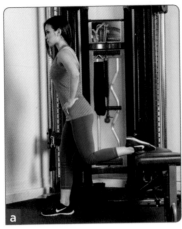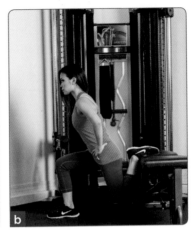

Figure 8.14 Bodyweight Bulgarian split squat: *(a)* starting position; *(b)* squat.

MUSCLES

Primary: quadriceps, gluteals

Secondary: hamstrings, adductors

MOVEMENT

1. Stand approximately 24 inches (60 cm) from a bench or a platform roughly 16 inches (40 cm) tall. Face away from the bench or platform.
2. Reach one leg back and rest the top of your foot flat against the platform.
3. With your hands on your hips, drop the knee of the back leg straight down in a controlled manner, making sure to keep the torso upright.
4. Graze the ground with the knee of the back leg and then return to the starting position.
5. After completing the desired number of repetitions on one side, switch legs and repeat.

TIPS

- Be careful not to put too much weight on the back leg. At the bottom of the movement, the shin of your front leg should be roughly vertical to the ground (or your knee should be approximately in line with your toe). Adjust your foot positioning if needed.
- Rest up to 45 seconds before switching legs and performing the repetitions on the other side.
- Don't let your hips shoot up first as you return to the starting position.
- Even advanced people lose their balance, so don't feel bad if you're squirmy as you perform your repetitions.

Variation 1: Dumbbell Bulgarian Split Squat

Perform the Bulgarian split squat while holding a dumbbell in each hand by your sides.

Variation 2: Goblet Bulgarian Split Squat

Perform the Bulgarian split squat while holding a dumbbell or kettlebell against your chest (figure 8.15).

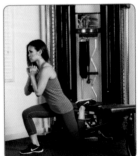

Figure 8.15 Goblet Bulgarian split squat.

HINGE PATTERN

The hinge pattern involves all the hip-dominant movements. Exercises in this category work the hamstrings the best and are good for the gluteals, but don't do as much for the quadriceps.

One of my go-to drills for teaching this pattern is the butt-tap drill (figure 8.16): Stand facing away from a wall, machine, or other vertical structure and try to tap it with your butt. When you do this, your hips should shoot back while the shins stay roughly vertical. You should have a slight bend in the knees, and the spine should stay in neutral the entire time.

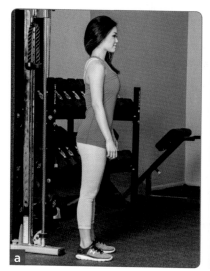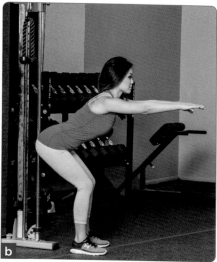

Figure 8.16 Butt-tap drill: *(a)* starting position; *(b)* hinge.

You can also wrap a resistance band around the hips and have a training partner gently pull it back to help train the movement pattern.

One of the biggest mistakes that beginner trainees make with the hinge pattern is to round at the low back. This action is dangerous and may lead to serious injury. If you're in doubt, be sure to spend extra time grooving the hinge pattern so that you look like figure 8.16.

The hinge pattern transfers to a number of movement patterns in sport, such as preparing for the vertical jump or playing defense in football.

Beginners should start with the pull-through and the Romanian deadlift before progressing to other variations.

CABLE PULL-THROUGH

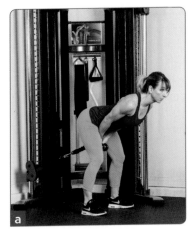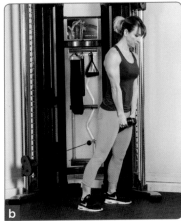

Figure 8.17 Cable pull-through: *(a)* starting position; *(b)* action.

MUSCLES

Primary: gluteals, hamstrings

Secondary: erectors

MOVEMENT

1. Secure a rope pulley attachment a few notches above the lowest setting on the machine.
2. Stand facing away from the pulley machine. Hold either side of the rope in your hands between your legs. Your palms should be facing up.
3. Take three big steps forward and lean forward.
4. Push the hips back while maintaining a soft bend in the knees, making sure to keep the chest up and back flat.
5. When you feel a stretch in your hamstrings, reverse the motion and push the hips through, squeezing the glutes at lockout.

TIPS

- At the bottom of the movement, the weight you're lifting off the cable pulley machine should not clank down against the weight stack. If this happens, you're too close to the machine, which will interfere with your ability to perform the movement with a full range of motion.
- To target more of the glutes and less of the low back, round the upper back and bend the knees more throughout the entire range of motion. Keeping your chin tucked may help as well.
- Maintain a forward lean for all repetitions to prevent the weight of the cable pulley machine from pulling you backward.
- Don't go so light that you aren't challenging your muscles; don't go so heavy that you don't feel it in your glutes or you're so off-balanced that you have to focus on not falling over.

Variation: Band Pull-Through

Perform the pull-through using a long resistance band looped around the bottom of a pole or squat rack.

BODYWEIGHT BACK EXTENSION

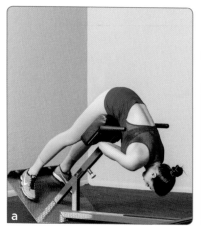 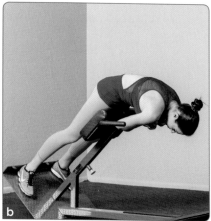

Figure 8.18 Bodyweight back extension: *(a)* starting position; *(b)* extension.

MUSCLES

Primary: hamstrings, gluteals

Secondary: erectors

MOVEMENT

1. Rest your hips against the padding of a back extension machine and secure your feet under the footpads or on the base.
2. Adjust the height of the padding so that the top of the padding rests right below your hip crease.
3. Bend over completely at the hips, with the toes pointed outward, and cross the arms over the chest. This is your starting position.
4. Keeping your chin tucked, actively round your upper back and push your upper back and push your hips into the padding as shown. You may appear not to be achieving full range of motion, but this is simply because you are in posterior pelvic tilt.
5. Squeeze the glutes to lockout and then reverse the motion.

TIPS

- You can perform the back extension on a glute–ham developer or a 45-degree hyperextension machine.
- Do not extend the spine as you rise up. Keep the spine in the same position throughout the range of motion. This exercise should really be called the hip extension, not the back extension.
- To target more of the low back and less of the gluteals, keep the toes pointed downward and lift your torso until your shoulders and head are in line with your hips and knees.
- Get a full stretch at the bottom of the movement.

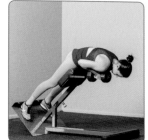

Variation: Dumbbell Back Extension

Perform the back extension while holding a dumbbell braced against the chest with both hands (figure 8.19).

Figure 8.19 Dumbbell back extension.

GOOD MORNING

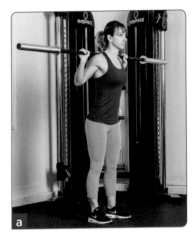 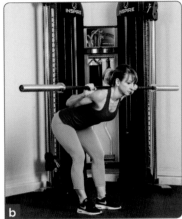

Figure 8.20   Good morning: *(a)* starting position; *(b)* action.

MUSCLES
Primary: hamstrings, erectors

Secondary: gluteals

MOVEMENT
1. Walk up to a barbell in a squat rack at approximately shoulder height.
2. Get under the barbell and unrack it so that it rests across your upper back.
3. Take two or three controlled steps back, away from the rack.
4. Position your feet at or slightly wider than shoulder-width apart.
5. Take in a deep breath and push the hips back while maintaining a soft bend in the knees, making sure to keep the chest up and back flat.
6. When you feel a stretch in your hamstrings, reverse the motion and push through the heels, squeezing the glutes at lockout. Exhale at the top of the repetition.

TIPS
- Use the high-bar position, not the low-bar position, for the good morning.
- Keep your shins roughly vertical to the ground throughout the movement. Don't let your knees come forward.
- Make sure you push through your heels, not your toes.
- Keep the spine in neutral and an arch in your back at the bottom of the movement.
- Go only as deep as you can go without rounding.

BODYWEIGHT REVERSE HYPEREXTENSION

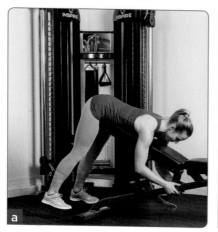 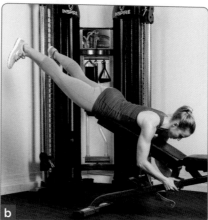

Figure 8.21 Bodyweight reverse hyperextension: *(a)* starting position; *(b)* hyperextension.

MUSCLES

Primary: hamstrings, gluteals

Secondary: erectors

MOVEMENT

1. Lie with the torso on top of a reverse hyperextension apparatus. If you don't have access to a reverse hyperextension apparatus, you can perform this exercise off an incline bench (as shown) or a stability ball. The legs should be pointing down.
2. Grab onto something sturdy such as the handles of the reverse hyperextension apparatus, the bar under the bench, or a solid structure. Extend the hips by swinging the legs back while pointing the toes out and spreading the legs. The spine should stay in neutral.
3. Squeeze the glutes at the top of the movement and then lower the legs to the starting position in a controlled manner.

TIPS

- Don't use too much momentum to finish your repetition. The movement should be strict and controlled.
- If you are using a reverse hyperextension apparatus, position the hip pad just above the pubic bone.
- Use a firm grip to stabilize yourself. Doing this can also help to activate other muscles.

Variation: Knee-Banded Reverse Hyperextension

Perform the reverse hyperextension with a miniband wrapped around the knees for increased glute activation. Alternatively, you can wrap a miniband around the midfoot.

BARBELL ROMANIAN DEADLIFT

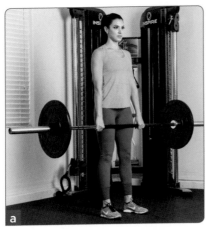 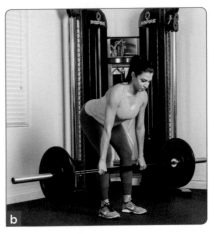

Figure 8.22 Barbell Romanian deadlift: *(a)* starting position; *(b)* action.

MUSCLES
Primary: hamstrings, erectors

Secondary: gluteals

MOVEMENT
1. Position your hands on a barbell resting on a rack at approximately knee height. Your grip should be just outside shoulder width.
2. Unrack the barbell by extending the hips while keeping the back flat.
3. Take two or three controlled steps back, away from the rack.
4. Position your feet approximately shoulder-width apart with your toes pointed forward.
5. Take in a deep breath and push the hips back while maintaining a soft bend in the knees, making sure to keep the chest up and back flat.
6. When the barbell moves past the knees and you feel a stretch in your hamstrings, reverse the motion and push through the heels while breathing out, squeezing the glutes at lockout. Exhale at the top of the repetition.

TIPS
- Imagine that someone is standing behind you with a rope around your hips and pulling back. This will help keep your back arched, keep your hips moving back, and prevent your knees from shooting forward.
- Maintain vertical shins (knees don't move forward) and a neutral spine as you descend, and keep the head and neck in neutral.
- Most people will be fine reversing the motion just below the knees, but those with incredible hamstring flexibility may need to get even greater range of motion to feel their hamstrings.
- Keep the barbell close to your body at all times. Don't let it drift away from you; it should skim your shins and thighs.
- You may find that grip becomes a limiting factor as you go heavier on this exercise. If that's the case, placing gym chalk on your hands or using a mixed grip (one hand overhand, one hand underhand) can help tremendously.

Variation 1: Dumbbell Romanian Deadlift
Perform the Romanian deadlift while holding dumbbells in front of you in both hands.

Variation 2: Dumbbell Single-Leg Romanian Deadlift

Perform the Romanian deadlift while holding a dumbbell on just one side of the body. With the other hand, hold onto something secure to brace yourself; this is a hamstring exercise, not a balance exercise. With the ipsilateral variation, you'll work the leg on the same side as the hand holding the dumbbell while kicking the other leg straight back; with the contralateral variation, you'll work the leg on the side opposite the hand holding the dumbbell (figure 8.23). The back leg should be in line with the torso.

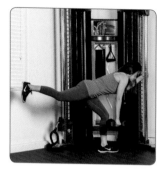

Figure 8.23 Dumbbell single-leg Romanian deadlift, contralateral variation.

AMERICAN DEADLIFT

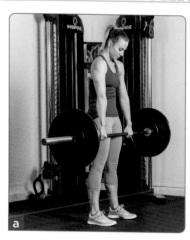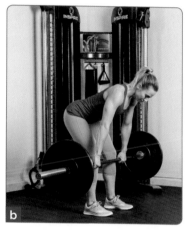

Figure 8.24 American deadlift: *(a)* starting position; *(b)* action.

MUSCLES

Primary: hamstrings, gluteals

Secondary: erectors

MOVEMENT

1. Position your hands on a barbell resting at approximately knee height on a rack. Your grip should be just outside shoulder width.
2. Unrack the barbell by extending the hips while keeping the back flat.
3. Take two or three controlled steps back, away from the rack.
4. Position your feet approximately shoulder-width apart with your toes pointed forward.
5. Take in a deep breath and push the hips back while maintaining a soft bend in the knees, making sure to keep the chest up and back flat.
6. When the barbell moves past the knees and you feel a stretch in your hamstrings, reverse the motion, push through the heels, and breathe out, rounding your upper back and squeezing the glutes at lockout.

(continued)

AMERICAN DEADLIFT *(continued)*

TIPS

- Unlike the Romanian deadlift, the American deadlift involves a posterior pelvic tilt and a strong glute squeeze at the top of the movement. This action helps to target the glutes more.
- Most people will be fine reversing the motion just below the knees, but those with incredible hamstring flexibility may need to get even greater range of motion to feel their hamstrings.
- Keep the barbell close to your body at all times. Don't let it drift away from you; it should skim your shins and thighs.
- You may find that grip becomes a limiting factor as you go heavier on this exercise. If that's the case, placing gym chalk on your hands or using a mixed grip (one hand overhand, one hand underhand) can help tremendously.

Variation: Snatch Grip American Deadlift

To perform the snatch grip American deadlift, grip the barbell several inches (cm) farther out so that the barbell can stay level with your hips at the beginning of the movement.

STIFF-LEGGED DEADLIFT

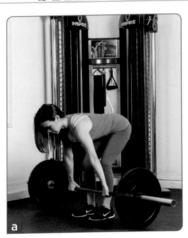 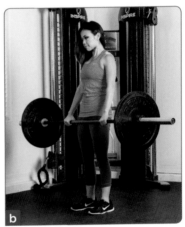

Figure 8.25 Stiff-legged deadlift: *(a)* starting position; *(b)* action.

MUSCLES

Primary: hamstrings, erectors

Secondary: gluteals

MOVEMENT

1. Load a barbell with plates and set it on the ground.
2. Step up to the barbell and position your feet approximately 6 to 10 inches (15 to 25 cm) apart and pointing forward. The barbell should intersect your midfeet.
3. Bend over while keeping the back in neutral and grab the barbell just outside your feet using either a double overhand grip or a mixed grip (one hand overhand, one hand underhand).
4. Take in a deep breath, generate tension in the lats, and lift the barbell off the ground with your hips high while keeping the barbell as close to your legs as possible throughout the duration of the lift.

5. At the top of the movement, roll the shoulders back and squeeze the glutes. Exhale and take in another deep breath.
6. Reverse the motion by pushing the hips back while maintaining a soft bend in the knees, making sure to keep the chest up and back flat.
7. Tap the barbell to the ground.

TIPS

- To prevent your shins from getting scraped and bloodied from the barbell, wear long pants or knee-high socks.
- If you find that grip is an issue, you can try using a mixed grip (one hand overhand, one hand underhand) or using gym chalk.
- If you're having trouble generating tension in your lats, think of squeezing pencils between your armpits.
- You can let the barbell drift away from you a little bit to get a better stretch in the hamstrings.
- If you can't deadlift 135 pounds (61 kg) yet (that would be a 45-pound [20 kg] plate on each side of the barbell), then use bumper plates; that way your range of motion remains the same. If you don't have access to bumper plates, you may find that setting your barbell down on risers or blocks a few inches (cm) high will help.

DEADLIFT

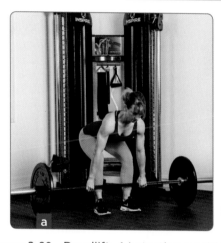
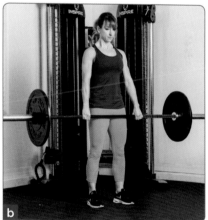

Figure 8.26 Deadlift: *(a)* starting position; *(b)* action.

MUSCLES

Primary: hamstrings, erectors

Secondary: gluteals

MOVEMENT

1. Load a barbell with plates and set it on the ground.
2. Step up to the barbell and position your feet approximately 6 to 10 inches (15 to 25 cm) apart and pointing forward. The barbell should intersect your midfeet.
3. Bend over and grab the barbell just outside your feet, using either a double overhand grip or a mixed grip (one hand overhand, one hand underhand).
4. Take in a deep breath, generate tension in the lats, and flatten the back.

(continued)

DEADLIFT *(continued)*

5. Lift the barbell off the ground while keeping the barbell as close to your shins as possible throughout the duration of the lift.
6. At the top of the movement, roll the shoulders back and squeeze the glutes. Exhale and take in another deep breath.
7. Reverse the motion by pushing the hips back while maintaining a soft bend in the knees, making sure to keep the chest up and back flat.
8. Set the barbell on the ground and take in another deep breath before doing another repetition.

TIPS

- To prevent your shins from getting scraped and bloodied from the barbell, wear long pants or knee-high socks.
- If you find that grip is an issue, you can try using a mixed grip (one hand overhand, one hand underhand) or using gym chalk.
- If you're having trouble generating tension in your lats, think of squeezing pencils between your armpits.
- Many beginner trainees make the mistake of trying to get their chest up by cranking their necks all the way back, but they still end up staying rounded over. Keep the chest up by thinking of showing the logo on your shirt to a person standing in front of you.
- If you can't deadlift 135 pounds (61 kg) yet (that would be a 45-pound [20 kg] plate on either side of the barbell), then use bumper plates; that way your range of motion remains the same. If you don't have access to bumper plates, you may find that setting your barbell on risers a few inches (cm) high will help.
- The method described here is a bottom-up setup, whereby you get down first before getting into position. Alternatively, you can perform this top down by bracing and generating tension in the lats while standing and then keeping the back flat while you reach down and grab the barbell.
- Don't let the hips shoot up as you start pulling the bar off the ground.

Variation 1: Kettlebell Deadlift

Perform the deadlift with a kettlebell. Position the kettlebell between your feet (figure 8.27).

Variation 2: Sumo Deadlift

Perform the deadlift with the feet in a wide sumo stance, toes pointed out at a 30- to 45-degree angle, and knees shoved out, not forward. You should drop your arms straight down from your shoulders and grab the barbell inside, not outside, the feet (figure 8.28). Your torso should stay more upright and the hips should be slightly lower than in the conventional deadlift. Be patient off the ground.

Variation 3: Trap-Bar Deadlift

Perform the trap-bar deadlift with your feet inside the trap bar positioned just inside shoulder-width apart and your arms holding the midpoint of each handle.

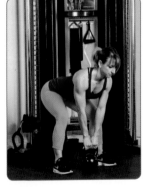

Figure 8.27 Kettlebell deadlift, starting position.

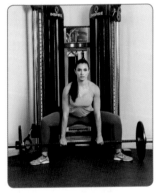

Figure 8.28 Sumo deadlift, starting position.

BRIDGE PATTERN

Bridge pattern movements include all bent-leg hip extension exercises. These are best for working the glutes, and they're decent at working the hamstrings. The movement involves pushing through the heels, extending the hips, and squeezing the glutes at lockout.

Typically, bridges are performed from a supine position on the floor, although alternatively the torso can be elevated onto a bench.

Bridge patterns entail horizontal loading and transfer uniquely to athletic performance, such as sprinting and horizontal jumping.

People of all anthropometries can become proficient at the bridge pattern. Beginners should master the bodyweight hip thrust first before adding load.

BARBELL GLUTE BRIDGE

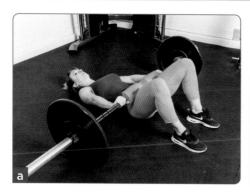
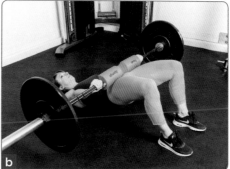

Figure 8.29 Barbell glute bridge: *(a)* starting position; *(b)* bridge.

MUSCLES

Primary: gluteals

Secondary: hamstrings, erectors

MOVEMENT

1. From a seated position on the ground with your legs out in front of you, roll a padded barbell over your legs and lie back into a supine position with the barbell at the hips just above the pubic bone.
2. Position the feet just outside shoulder width, flatten the lumbar spine, and place the heels on the ground with the knees at approximately a 90-degree angle.
3. With your hands on the barbell holding it in place on the hips, extend the hips and raise the barbell off the floor, pushing through the heels.
4. Achieve full hip extension and squeeze the glutes at lockout.
5. Lower the barbell to the ground in a controlled manner.

(continued)

BARBELL GLUTE BRIDGE   *(continued)*

TIPS

- Some people feel their glutes activating better with a wide stance with their feet, whereas others prefer a hip-width stance. Experiment with both methods and find what works best for you.
- Make sure to keep your ribs down and don't arch your back during your repetitions.
- If you find that your range of motion is limited by the plates on the barbell touching the ground (with bumper plates or 45-pound [20 kg] plates), you may see better results using 25-pound (11 kg) plates and having a training partner deadlift the barbell onto your lap.

Variation 1: Barbell Knee-Banded Glute Bridge

Perform the glute bridge with a miniband wrapped around the knees.

Variation 2: Bodyweight Glute Bridge

Perform the glute bridge with just your body weight (no added load).

Variation 3: Knee-Banded Bodyweight Glute Bridge

Perform the knee-banded bodyweight glute bridge with a miniband wrapped around the knees.

Variation 4: Dumbbell Glute Bridge

Perform the glute bridge with a dumbbell held horizontally across the hips.

Variation 5: Dumbbell Knee-Banded Glute Bridge

Perform the dumbbell glute bridge with a miniband wrapped around the knees.

SINGLE-LEG GLUTE BRIDGE

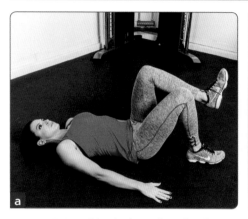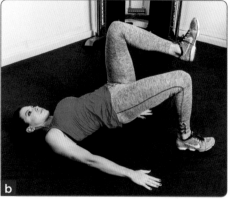

Figure 8.30 Single-leg glute bridge: *(a)* starting position; *(b)* bridge.

MUSCLES

Primary: gluteals

Secondary: hamstrings, erectors

MOVEMENT

1. From a seated position on the ground with your legs out in front of you, lie back into a supine position.
2. Flatten the lumbar spine and center one heel on the ground with the knee at approximately a 90-degree angle. The other leg can be fully extended, hovering just above the ground, or bent.
3. Extend the hips, pushing through the heel of the working leg.
4. Achieve full hip extension and squeeze the glutes at lockout.
5. Lower the hips to the ground in a controlled manner. After completing repetitions on one leg, switch to the other leg.

TIP

Make sure to keep your ribs down and don't arch your back when performing your repetitions.

FEET-ELEVATED GLUTE BRIDGE

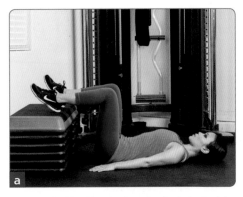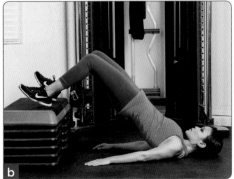

Figure 8.31   Feet-elevated glute bridge: *(a)* starting position; *(b)* bridge.

MUSCLES

Primary: gluteals

Secondary: hamstrings, erectors

MOVEMENT

1. From a seated position on the ground with a weight bench, step, or platform in front of you, lie back into a supine position.
2. Position the feet just outside shoulder width, flatten the lumbar spine, and place the heels on the bench, step, or platform with the knees at approximately a 90-degree angle.
3. Extend the hips, pushing through the heels.
4. Achieve full hip extension and squeeze the glutes at lockout.
5. Lower the hips to the ground in a controlled manner.

TIPS

- The feet-elevated glute bridge is a great way to take the quadriceps out of the equation, especially for those who feel the quads overpower during hip thrusts.
- You can make fists with your hands and dig your elbows into the ground to prevent your arms and hands from flailing about.

Variation: Knee-Banded Feet-Elevated Glute Bridge

Perform the feet-elevated glute bridge with a miniband wrapped around the knees.

BARBELL HIP THRUST

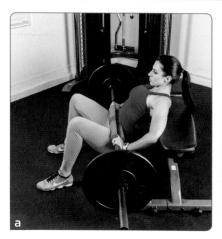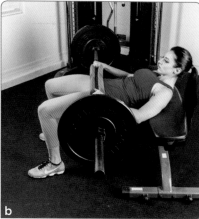

Figure 8.32 Barbell hip thrust: *(a)* starting position; *(b)* hip thrust.

MUSCLES

Primary: gluteals

Secondary: hamstrings, quadriceps, adductors

MOVEMENT

1. Sit on the floor with the legs extended, leaning back against a bench approximately 14 inches (36 cm) tall.
2. Roll a padded barbell over the hips just above the pubic bone.
3. Position the feet just outside shoulder width, place the heels on the ground with the knees at approximately a 90-degree angle, and line up the bench just under the shoulder blades.
4. With your hands on the barbell to hold it in place on the hips, take in a big breath, brace the core, extend the hips, and raise the barbell off the floor, pushing through the heels.
5. Achieve full hip extension and squeeze the glutes at lockout.
6. Lower the barbell to the ground in a controlled manner. Exhale and take in another deep breath before completing another repetition.

TIPS

- Depending on the length of your torso, you may find that a bench height of 13 to 19 inches (33 to 48 cm) tall suits you better.
- Ensure that your shins are roughly vertical at the top of the movement. If your feet are too far out in front of you, you may feel your hamstrings working more than your glutes; if your feet are too close to you, you may feel your quads working.
- Keep the chin tucked, ribs down, and eyes forward throughout the movement. Strength coach Ben Bruno tells his clients to keep their eyes in front of them where the wall meets the ceiling.
- Use a weight heavy enough that you can feel your glutes activating. If you go too heavy, you may find that your chest flares up, your neck cranks back, you can't reach full lockout, and you feel the movement in your low back rather than in your glutes. Scale back the weight if necessary.

(continued)

BARBELL GLUTE BRIDGE *(continued)*

Variation 1: Knee-Banded Barbell Hip Thrust

Perform the barbell hip thrust with a miniband wrapped around the knees.

Variation 2: Bodyweight Hip Thrust

Perform the hip thrust with no weight, fists clenched, and elbows digging into the bench.

Variation 3: Knee-Banded Bodyweight Hip Thrust

Perform the bodyweight hip thrust with a miniband wrapped around the knees.

Variation 4: Dumbbell Hip Thrust

Perform the hip thrust while holding a dumbbell horizontally across the hips.

Variation 5: Knee-Banded Dumbbell Hip Thrust

Perform the dumbbell hip thrust with a miniband wrapped around the knees.

Variation 6: Hip-Banded Hip Thrust

Perform the hip thrust with a long resistance band anchored to the ground on either side of you and the band across your hips. This exercise will be easiest using the hooks of a Hip Thruster, but it can also be done with dumbbells crisscrossed against each other or with the pegs of a power rack. Don't be afraid to get creative with this exercise.

Variation 7: Hip- and Knee-Banded Hip Thrust

Perform the hip thrust with a miniband wrapped around the knees and a resistance band across the hips, anchored to the ground on either side of you.

BODYWEIGHT SINGLE-LEG HIP THRUST

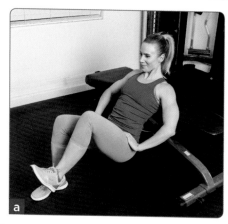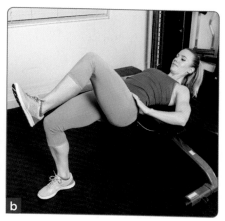

Figure 8.33 Bodyweight single-leg hip thrust: *(a)* starting position; *(b)* hip thrust.

MUSCLES

Primary: gluteals

Secondary: hamstrings, quadriceps, adductors

MOVEMENT

1. Sit on the floor with the legs extended. Lean back against a bench approximately 14 inches (36 cm) tall.
2. Center one heel on the ground with the knee at approximately a 90-degree angle. The other leg can be fully extended or slightly bent, hovering just above the ground. Line up the bench just under the shoulder blades.
3. Take in a big breath, brace the core, and extend the hips off the floor, pushing through the heel.
4. Achieve full hip extension and squeeze the glutes at lockout.
5. Lower the hips to the ground in a controlled manner. Exhale and take in another deep breath before completing another repetition.
6. After you have performed all repetitions on one side, switch legs and perform the same number of repetitions on the other side.

TIPS

- The major cues for the single-leg hip thrust are the same as those for the bilateral hip thrust: Keep the chin tucked, ribs down, and eyes forward; achieve full hip extension; and squeeze the glutes at lockout.
- Work your weaker leg first and then do the same number of repetitions with the stronger leg.

Variation 1: Dumbbell Single-Leg Hip Thrust

Perform the single-leg hip thrust with a dumbbell braced against the hip of the working leg.

Variation 2: Bodyweight Single-Leg Knee-Banded Hip Thrust

Perform the bodyweight single-leg hip thrust with a miniband wrapped just above the knees.

FROG PUMP

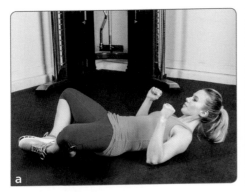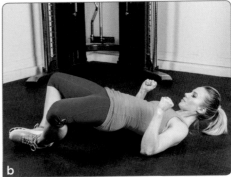

Figure 8.34 Frog pump: *(a)* starting position; *(b)* action.

MUSCLES

Primary: gluteals

Secondary: hamstrings

MOVEMENT

1. Lie in a supine position with the heels pressed together.
2. Flatten the lumbar spine, tuck the chin, and place the elbows on the ground, hands in fists.
3. Extend the hips to full hip extension and squeeze the glutes at lockout.
4. Lower the hips to the ground.

TIPS

- These repetitions do not need to be slow and controlled. Go for the pump. But you may want to pause at the top of each repetition and give the glutes an extra squeeze.
- Rather than placing the elbows on the ground, you can alternatively place your palms on the ground.

Variation: Dumbbell Frog Pump

Perform the frog pump with a dumbbell braced against the hips.

BODYWEIGHT QUADRUPED HIP EXTENSION

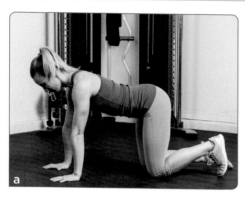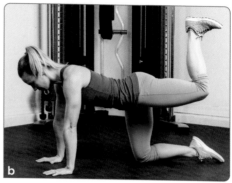

Figure 8.35 Bodyweight quadruped hip extension: *(a)* starting position; *(b)* hip extension.

MUSCLES

Primary: gluteals

Secondary: hamstrings

MOVEMENT

1. Assume a quadruped position on your hands and knees. Your knees should be directly below your hips, and your hands should be directly below your shoulders.
2. While keeping the hips as square as possible, lift one leg toward the ceiling while keeping the knee bent.
3. Squeeze the glutes at the top of the movement.
4. Lower the working leg to the ground in a controlled manner. After completing your repetitions, switch to the other side.

TIPS

- The knee of the working leg should not touch the ground between repetitions.
- Avoid excessive arching of the low back.

Variation 1: Knee-Banded Quadruped Hip Extension

Perform the quadruped hip extension with a miniband wrapped just above the knees.

Variation 2: Ankle Weight Quadruped Hip Extension

Perform the quadruped hip extension with an ankle weight wrapped around the ankle of the working leg.

LATERAL ROTARY

Lateral rotary exercises are an often-overlooked aspect of a training program. The movement pattern includes lateral movements that involve hip abduction and rotary movements that involve hip external rotation.

Lateral rotary movements work the parts of the glutes that aren't worked during hip extension. The frontal plane movements target the upper gluteals (upper division of the gluteus maximus and the gluteus medius), and the rotational movements work the entire gluteus maximus in addition to the hip external rotator. These exercises are important not only for optimal glute development but also for improved mechanics and prevention of dangerous movements such as knee valgus.

These exercises are low impact, so performing a large number of repetitions won't tax your body as, say, deadlifts would. Lateral rotary exercises are typically incorporated into the end of a workout.

LATERAL WALK

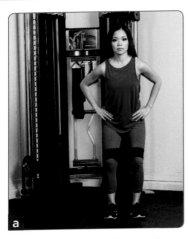 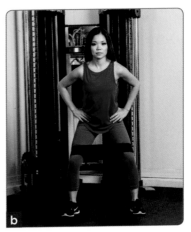

Figure 8.36 Lateral walk: *(a)* starting position; *(b)* walk.

MUSCLES
Primary: gluteals

MOVEMENT
1. Stand with a miniband placed either above or below the knees. Position the feet approximately shoulder-width apart.
2. With the hands on the hips and a soft bend in the knees, push off the lateral edges of the grounded foot and take a big step out to the side with the other leg.
3. Complete the desired number of repetitions and then repeat on the other side.

TIPS
- The size of the step you take depends on the tension in the miniband and the target number of repetitions.
- You may find your glutes working more when you bend over slightly at the hips versus staying upright.

MONSTER WALK

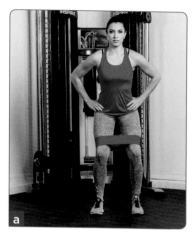 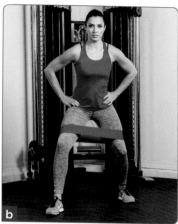

Figure 8.37 Monster walk: *(a)* starting position; *(b)* walk.

MUSCLES

Primary: gluteals

MOVEMENT

1. Stand with a miniband placed either above or below the knees. Position the feet approximately shoulder-width apart.
2. With the hands on the hips and a soft bend in the knees, push off the lateral edge of the grounded foot and take a big step forward with the other leg.
3. Step off the heel of the front foot and take another step forward.
4. Complete the desired number of repetitions.

TIPS

- The size of the step you take depends on the tension in the miniband and the target number of repetitions.
- You can up the ante of this movement by coming out onto the lateral edges of the front foot and pushing that knee out with each step.

BODYWEIGHT SIDE-LYING CLAMSHELL

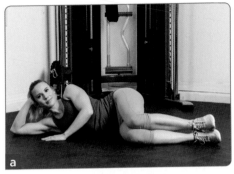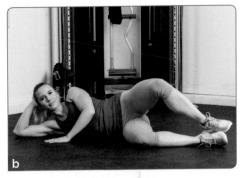

Figure 8.38 Bodyweight side-lying clamshell: *(a)* starting position; *(b)* action.

MUSCLES
Primary: gluteals

MOVEMENT
1. Lie on your side with the feet stacked together. The hips should be at approximately a 135-degree angle and the legs at approximately a 90-degree angle.
2. With the heels pressed together, rotate the top knee up.
3. Lower the top knee back to the starting position. After finishing your repetitions, switch to the other side.

TIPS
- You can rest the bottom arm against the floor for balance, or you can use it to prop up your head. You can rest the hand of the top arm against the floor or palpate the working glute.
- Some people feel their glutes activating better with the knees closer to their bodies; others feel it better farther away. Tinker with different angles of the hip and knee to find what works best for you.

Variation: Band Side-Lying Clamshell
Perform the side-lying clamshell with a miniband positioned just above the knees.

BODYWEIGHT SIDE-LYING HIP ABDUCTION

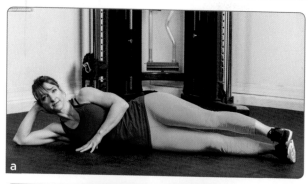

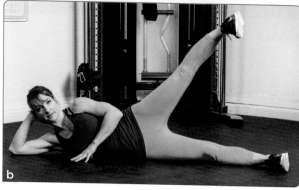

Figure 8.39 Bodyweight side-lying hip abduction: *(a)* starting position; *(b)* hip abduction.

MUSCLES

Primary: gluteals

MOVEMENT

1. Lie on your side with the feet stacked together and the legs fully extended.
2. Lift the top leg as high as it will go, turning the heel slightly outward.
3. Lower the top leg to the starting position. After completing your repetitions, switch to the other side.

TIP

You can rest the bottom arm against the floor for balance, or you can use it to prop up your head. You can rest the hand of the top arm against the floor or palpate the working glute.

Variation: Ankle Weight Side-Lying Hip Abduction

Perform the side-lying hip abduction with an ankle weight wrapped around the ankle of the working leg.

SEATED BAND HIP ABDUCTION

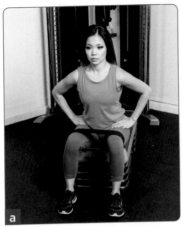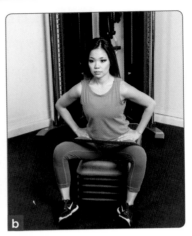

Figure 8.40 Seated band hip abduction: *(a)* starting position; *(b)* hip abduction.

MUSCLES
Primary: upper gluteals

MOVEMENT
1. Wrap a miniband above or below the knees and sit on a bench or box 12 to 16 inches (30 to 40 cm) tall. Plant the feet on the floor approximately shoulder-width apart.
2. Leaning forward with the chest up and the low back flat, spread the knees apart, rolling onto the outer edges of the feet.
3. Return the knees to the starting position.

TIP
Try this movement upright and when leaning back in the seated position. Perform the variation that works your glutes the best. If you feel your glutes activating roughly equally in all three positions, incorporate all three into your workout.

Variation: Seated Machine Hip Abduction
Perform the seated hip abduction on a hip abduction machine. You can do this while sitting upright or leaning forward, keeping the chest up and the low back flat.

STANDING BAND HIP ABDUCTION

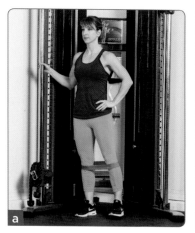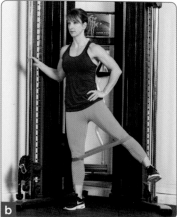

Figure 8.41 Standing band hip abduction: *(a)* starting position; *(b)* hip abduction.

MUSCLES

Primary: upper gluteals

MOVEMENT

1. Stand next to a power rack or something sturdy to hold for balance with a miniband wrapped above or below the knees.
2. Keeping the weight of the body on one foot, extend the other leg out to the side, turning the toe of the working leg in slightly.
3. Return the working leg to the starting position. Switch to the other side.

TIPS

- Lead the movement with the heel to feel better activation of the upper glutes.
- The upper glutes of the grounded leg work hard to stabilize the body, so rest for 10 to 20 seconds before switching to the other side.

Variation 1: Standing Cable Hip Abduction

Perform the standing cable hip abduction with a handle pulley wrapped around the ankle and attached to the lowest setting on a cable machine.

Variation 2: Standing Ankle Weight Hip Abduction

Perform the standing ankle weight hip abduction with an ankle weight wrapped around the ankle of the working leg.

STANDING BAND HIP HINGE ABDUCTION

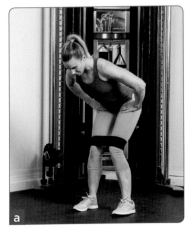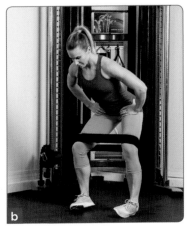

Figure 8.42 Standing hip hinge abduction: *(a)* starting position; *(b)* hip abduction.

MUSCLES

Primary: gluteals

MOVEMENT

1. Stand with a miniband wrapped above or below the knees and the feet approximately shoulder-width apart.
2. Hinge at the hips with a slight bend in the knees. Keep the chest up and the low back flat as though you're performing the Romanian deadlift.
3. With the hands on the hips, spread the knees apart, rolling onto the outer edges of the feet.
4. Return to the starting position.

TIP

The hips should shoot back, and the knees should not travel forward.

FIRE HYDRANT

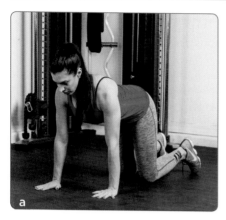 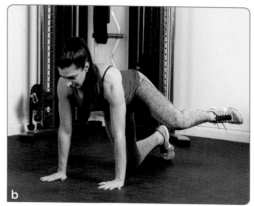

Figure 8.43 Fire hydrant: *(a)* starting position; *(b)* action.

MUSCLES

Primary: gluteals

MOVEMENT

1. Assume a quadruped position on your hands and knees. Your knees should be directly below your hips, and your hands should be directly below your shoulders.
2. While keeping the hips as square as possible, lift one leg out to the side while keeping the knee bent.
3. Lower the working leg back to the ground in a controlled manner. After completing your repetitions, switch to the other side.

TIP

Avoid excess movement in the torso and ensure that only the working leg is moving.

Variation 1: Knee-Banded Fire Hydrant

Perform the fire hydrant with a miniband wrapped above the knees.

Variation 2: Ankle Weight Fire Hydrant

Perform the fire hydrant with an ankle weight wrapped around the ankle of the working leg.

UPPER-BODY PUSH

Upper-body push movements work the pressing muscles, which include the pecs, front delts, and triceps.

The exercises can be further divided into upper-body vertical push and upper-body horizontal push. The vertical exercises work the delts more, and the horizontal exercises work the pecs more, but there is a good deal of overlap.

Although men in particular like to perform upper-body push exercises, women should also include these in their training programs for a strong and balanced body.

Beginners should start with the incline push-up and the dumbbell bench press.

BARBELL MILITARY PRESS

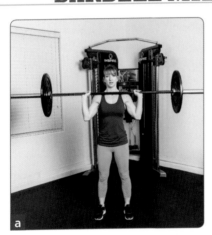 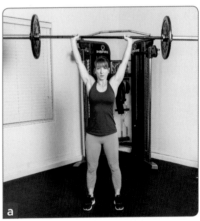

Figure 8.44   Barbell military press: *(a)* starting position; *(b)* press.

MUSCLES
Primary: deltoids
Secondary: triceps, upper trapezius

MOVEMENT
1. Walk up to a barbell in a rack at approximately shoulder height.
2. Grab the barbell with both hands just outside shoulder-width apart. The barbell should sit comfortably in the groove of the palms.
3. Unrack the barbell and take two or three controlled steps back. Position the feet approximately shoulder-width apart. Point the toes straight forward or slightly out.
4. Beginning with the bar at the top of the sternum, take in a deep breath, squeeze the glutes, and press the barbell overhead. The elbows should stay tucked close to the body.
5. Lock out the elbows at the top of the movement. Make sure you stand tall and push the head through.
6. Lower the barbell to the sternum in a controlled manner. Exhale and take in another deep breath before completing another repetition.

TIPS
- At the top of the movement, stand tall and push the head through.
- Be careful not to use momentum to press the barbell overhead. This is the military press, not the push press.

Variation: Dumbbell Military Press

Perform the military press while holding a dumbbell in each hand. The elbows should be at approximately a 45-degree angle to the body, and the dumbbells should be in line with the upper arms.

BARBELL PUSH PRESS

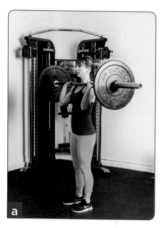 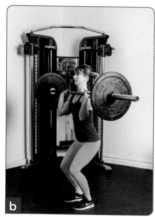 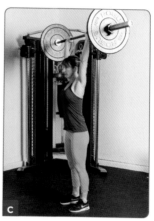

Figure 8.45 Barbell push press: *(a)* starting position; *(b)* flex knees and hips; *(c)* press.

MUSCLES

Primary: deltoids

Secondary: triceps, upper trapezius, quadriceps

MOVEMENT

1. Walk up to a barbell in a rack at approximately shoulder height.
2. Grab the barbell with both hands just outside shoulder-width apart. The barbell should sit comfortably in the groove of the palms.
3. Unrack the barbell and take two or three controlled steps back. Position the feet approximately shoulder-width apart. Point the toes straight forward or slightly out.
4. Beginning with the bar at the top of the sternum, take in a deep breath and slightly flex the knees and hips. The torso should stay upright.
5. Immediately press the bar up in an explosive motion by extending the knees and pushing through the heels.
6. Lower the barbell, flexing the knees as the barbell touches the sternum. Exhale and take in another deep breath before completing another repetition.

TIPS

- At the top of the movement, stand tall and push the head through.
- Be careful not to let the hips shoot back too much. The knees should travel forward.

Variation: Dumbbell Push Press

Perform the push press while holding a dumbbell in each hand. The elbows should be at approximately a 45-degree angle to the body, and the dumbbells should be in line with the upper arms.

STANDING LANDMINE PRESS

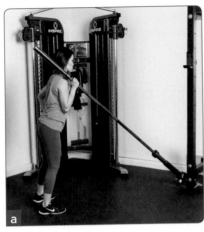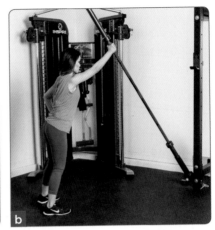

Figure 8.46 Standing landmine press: *(a)* starting position; *(b)* press.

MUSCLES

Primary: deltoids

Secondary: upper pecs, triceps, upper trapezius

MOVEMENT

1. Place a barbell in a landmine position by wrapping a towel around one end and wedging it into a corner. Alternatively, you can position a barbell into a landmine device.
2. Keeping the core in a neutral position, hold the other end of the barbell in one hand resting a few inches (cm) above the upper pec near the armpit. The elbow of the working arm should be approximately 30 degrees away from the body.
3. As you press the barbell up, lean slightly into the bar and fully extend the arm. The arm should be approximately 110 degrees relative to the body.
4. Lower the barbell in a controlled manner. After finishing your repetitions, switch to the other side.

TIPS

- When adding load, use smaller plates to prevent the weights from getting in the way of movement execution.
- Keep the core in a neutral position throughout the entire movement.
- Don't let the lower back extend as you press the barbell up.

Variation: Half-Kneeling Landmine Press

Perform the landmine press from a half-kneeling position. The knee and hip should be in a 90-degree position.

BARBELL BENCH PRESS

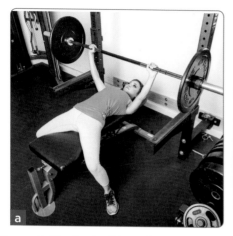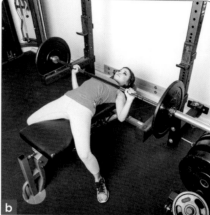

Figure 8.47 Barbell bench press: *(a)* starting position; *(b)* press.

MUSCLES

Primary: pectorals

Secondary: anterior deltoids, triceps

MOVEMENT

1. Lie flat on a bench with the feet on the floor. Position the body so that the barbell is directly above the mouth.
2. Using an overhand grip just outside shoulder-width, unrack the barbell and position it above the upper chest. The arms should be locked, and the wrists should be straight.
3. Take in a deep breath and lower the barbell to the midchest in a controlled manner.
4. Press the barbell back up until the arms are fully extended, pushing it back toward your face. Think of creating an arc with the barbell. Exhale.

TIPS

- Don't let your elbows flare out as you press the barbell up. They should stay at approximately a 45-degree angle to the body. Think of making an arrow with the arms and the body, not a T.
- Don't let the barbell drift away from you as you press it up. This deviation creates an inefficient bar path and makes the movement more difficult.
- The butt should not lift off the bench at any point during the movement.
- Think of pulling your chest up to the bar rather than simply bringing it down toward you. This approach helps create tension throughout the upper body.
- To lift more weight, create an arch in the back, bring the feet close to the body, and turn the heels out. This position will help create better leg drive and decrease the range of motion that the bar has to travel.

Variation: Dumbbell Bench Press

Perform the bench press while holding a dumbbell in each hand. The elbows should be at approximately a 45-degree angle to the body, and the dumbbells should be in line with the upper arms.

BARBELL FLOOR PRESS

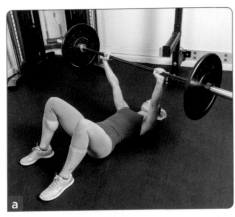 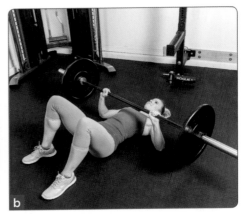

Figure 8.48 Barbell floor press: *(a)* starting position; *(b)* press.

MUSCLES

Primary: pectorals

Secondary: anterior deltoids, triceps

MOVEMENT

1. Lie flat on the floor. Place the heels on the ground with the knees at approximately a 90-degree angle and position the body under the barbell.
2. Using an overhand grip just outside shoulder width, position the barbell above the upper chest. The arms should be locked, and the wrists should be straight.
3. Take in a deep breath and lower the barbell in a controlled manner.
4. Tap the elbows to the ground and then press the barbell back up until the arms are fully extended, pushing it back toward your face. Think of creating an arc with the barbell. Exhale and take in another deep breath before completing another repetition.

TIPS

- Don't let your elbows flare out as you press up the barbell. They should stay at approximately a 45-degree angle to the body. Think of making an arrow with the arms and the body, not a T.
- Don't let the barbell drift away from you as you press it up. This deviation creates an inefficient bar path and makes the movement more difficult.
- Think of pulling your chest up to the bar rather than simply bringing it down toward you. This approach helps create tension throughout the upper body.

Variation: Dumbbell Floor Press

Perform the floor press while holding a dumbbell in each hand. The elbows should be at approximately a 45-degree angle to the body, and the dumbbells should be in line with the upper arms.

BARBELL INCLINE PRESS

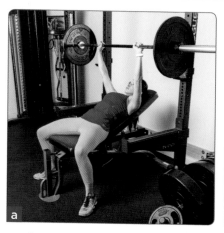 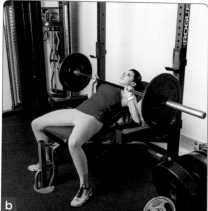

Figure 8.49 Barbell incline press: *(a)* starting position; *(b)* press.

MUSCLES

Primary: pectorals, anterior deltoids

Secondary: triceps

MOVEMENT

1. Sit on an incline bench positioned at approximately a 45-degree angle.
2. Using an overhand grip just outside shoulder width, unrack the barbell and position it above the upper chest. The arms should be locked, and the wrists should be straight.
3. Take in a deep breath and lower the barbell in a controlled manner.
4. Touch the barbell on the upper chest and then press the barbell back up until the arms are fully extended, pushing it back toward your face.
5. Exhale and take in another deep breath before completing another repetition.

TIPS

- With the incline press, the barbell should touch your chest higher than it does for the flat barbell bench press.
- The elbows can flare out more than they do for the barbell bench press.

Variation: Dumbbell Incline Press

Perform the dumbbell incline press with a dumbbell in each hand.

CLOSE-GRIP BENCH PRESS

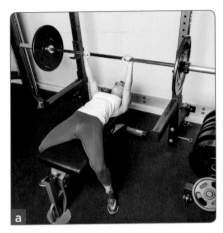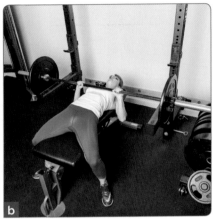

Figure 8.50 Close-grip bench press: *(a)* starting position; *(b)* press.

MUSCLES

Primary: pectorals, triceps

Secondary: anterior deltoids

MOVEMENT

1. Lie flat on a bench with the feet on the floor. Position the body so that the barbell is directly above the mouth.
2. Using an overhand grip just inside shoulder width, unrack the barbell and position it above the upper chest. The arms should be locked, and the wrists should be straight.
3. Take in a deep breath and lower the barbell to the midchest in a controlled manner.
4. Press the barbell back up until the arms are fully extended, pushing it back toward your face. Think of creating an arc with the barbell.
5. Exhale and take in another deep breath before completing another repetition.

TIPS

- Your grip for the close-grip bench press should be about one hand-width narrower per side than for it is the regular flat bench press.
- Don't let your elbows flare out as you press the barbell up. They should stay at approximately a 45-degree angle to the body. Think of making an arrow, not a T, with the arms and the body.
- Don't let the barbell drift away from you as you press it up. This deviation creates an inefficient bar path and makes the movement more difficult.
- The butt should not lift off the bench at any point during the movement.
- Think of pulling your chest up to the bar rather than simply bringing it down toward you. This approach will help create tension throughout the upper body.
- To lift more weight, create an arch in the back, bring the feet in close to the body, and turn the heels out. This position will create better leg drive and decrease the range of motion that the bar has to travel.

BODYWEIGHT PUSH-UP

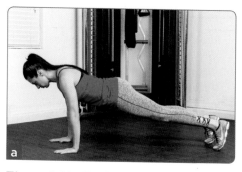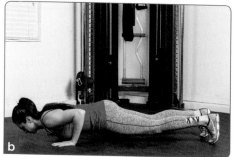

Figure 8.51 Bodyweight push-up: *(a)* starting position; *(b)* push-up.

MUSCLES

Primary: pectorals

Secondary: anterior deltoids, triceps

MOVEMENT

1. Start in a plank position with the arms extended and the body in a straight line. Place the hands just outside shoulder width on the floor.
2. Keeping the head, neck, and spine in a neutral position, lower the chest to the floor, and touch the chest to the ground. The upper arms should be fairly tucked at a 30- to 45-degree angle relative to the torso, and the body should be kept in a straight line.
3. Reverse the motion by pushing the body back up to the starting position.

TIPS

- At no point during the movement should the hips sag. Keep the glutes squeezed and posteriorly tilt the pelvis.
- Most people want to have the elbows pointing straight out to the sides and the body in a T shape. Think of making an arrow instead.
- Maintain good neutral spinal posture. Don't flex the upper back or anteriorly tilt the pelvis.
- Don't reach with the head during the movement.

Variation 1: Incline Push-Up

Perform this movement with arms elevated on a bench (figure 8.52) or another elevated, sturdy surface such as the pins of a power rack. The higher the incline is, the easier the movement will be.

Variation 2: Narrow-Width Push-Up

Perform a push-up with the hands just inside shoulder width or narrower.

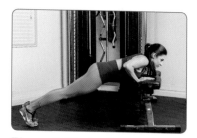

Figure 8.52 Incline push-up.

UPPER-BODY PULL

Upper-body pull movements work the pulling muscles: the lats, midtraps, rhomboids, and biceps.

Performing a full bodyweight chin-up is probably one of the most exciting accomplishments of a woman's ventures in the gym. If this is something that you're striving to accomplish, know that it's entirely possible to do it with repeated practice.

You should strive to include a similar volume of upper-body pushing and pulling movements in a well-rounded training program. Therefore, you'll typically find at least one upper-body push exercise and one upper-body pull exercise in every full-body workout.

Beginners should start with the lat pulldown and the seated row.

BODYWEIGHT CHIN-UP

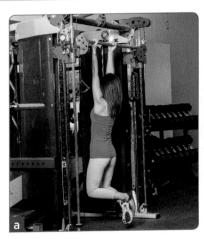 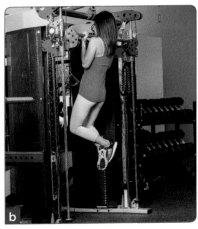

Figure 8.53 Bodyweight chin-up: *(a)* starting position; *(b)* chin-up.

MUSCLES
Primary: lats, midtraps, rhomboids

Secondary: biceps

MOVEMENT
1. Begin with an underhand grip on a bar with the hands approximately shoulder-width apart. The arms should be fully extended, and the body should be in a dead hang position.
2. Using the lats, pull the torso up to the bar while keeping the elbows close to the body.
3. Touch the sternum to the bar and then lower the body in a controlled manner until the arms are fully extended.

TIPS
- Don't use excessive body language when performing this movement. There should be no kipping motion, and the legs should not flail about.
- Instead of reaching with your neck, think of trying to touch your chest to the bar.
- You can keep the legs extended or cross them at the ankles while performing this movement.

- Tinker with grip width to find what feels best for you. Some people like a narrow grip, with the hands approximately 6 inches (15 cm) apart, whereas others prefer to have the hands just outside shoulder width.

Variation 1: Band-Assisted Chin-Up

Perform the chin-up with a long resistance band looped around the bar and under the feet (figure 8.54).

Variation 2: Weighted Chin-Up

Perform the chin-up with a plate or dumbbell held between the legs or hanging off a weight belt.

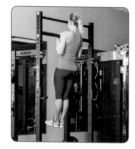

Figure 8.54 Band-assisted chin-up.

BODYWEIGHT PULL-UP

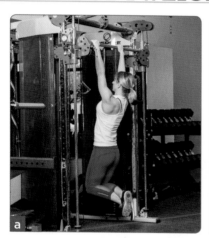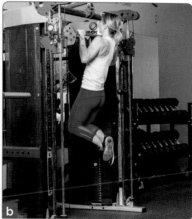

Figure 8.55 Bodyweight pull-up: (a) starting position; (b) pull-up.

MUSCLES

Primary: lats, midtraps, rhomboids

Secondary: biceps

MOVEMENT

1. Begin with an overhand grip on a bar with the hands approximately shoulder-width apart. The arms should be fully extended, and the body should be in a dead hang position.
2. Using the lats, pull the torso up to the bar while keeping the elbows close to the body.
3. Touch the sternum to the bar and then lower the body in a controlled manner until the arms are fully extended.

TIPS

- Don't use excessive body language when performing this movement. There should be no kipping motion, and the legs should not flail about.
- Instead of reaching with your neck, think of trying to touch your chest to the bar.
- You can keep the legs extended or cross them at the ankles while performing this movement.

(continued)

- Tinker with grip width to find what feels best for you. Some people like a narrow grip with the hands approximately 6 inches (15 cm) apart, whereas others prefer to have the hands just outside shoulder width.

Variation 1: Band-Assisted Pull-Up

Perform the pull-up with a long resistance band looped around the bar and under the feet.

Variation 2: Weighted Pull-Up

Perform the pull-up with a plate or dumbbell held between the legs or hanging off a weight belt.

Variation 3: Bodyweight Neutral-Grip Pull-Up

Begin with a neutral grip (palms facing in) on a bar with the hands approximately shoulder-width apart. The arms should be fully extended, and the body should be in a dead hang position. Perform the pull-up, touch the sternum to the bar, and then lower the body in a controlled manner until the arms are fully extended. This variation can be performed as a band-assisted pull-up or a weighted pull-up as well.

LAT PULLDOWN

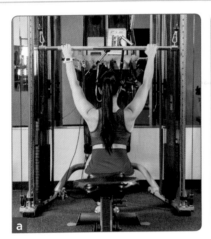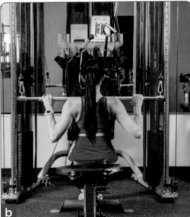

Figure 8.56 Lat pulldown: *(a)* starting position; *(b)* pulldown.

MUSCLES

Primary: lats

Secondary: biceps

MOVEMENT

1. Assume an overhand grip on the wide bar of a lat pulldown machine with the hands wider than shoulder-width apart.
2. Sit on the seat and slide the legs under the kneepads to prevent the resistance of the bar from lifting the body up.
3. Keeping the chest up, pull the bar down until it touches the collarbone by drawing the upper arms down and back.
4. Return the bar to the starting position in a controlled manner until the arms are fully extended.

- At no point should the shoulders roll forward or the upper back round.
- Don't lean back too much when performing this exercise. The torso should stay relatively upright throughout the movement.

Variation 1: V-Handle Lat Pulldown

Perform the lat pulldown with the V-handle attached to the pulley machine.

Variation 2: Wide-Grip Lat Pulldown

Perform the lat pulldown with the hands gripping the bar just outside shoulder-width apart.

TALL-KNEELING SINGLE-ARM CABLE PULL-IN

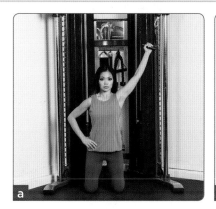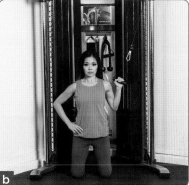

Figure 8.57 Tall-kneeling single-arm cable pull-in: *(a)* starting position; *(b)* pull-in.

MUSCLES

Primary: lats

Secondary: biceps

MOVEMENT

1. Grasp a handle attached to the top notch of a pulley machine. Assume a tall-kneeling position so that the working arm is fully extended at approximately a 135-degree angle relative to the body.
2. Keeping the torso upright, contract the lat of the working side and pull in the handle with the working arm until the elbow is parallel to the torso.
3. Return the handle to the starting position in a controlled manner until the arm is fully extended.
4. After completing all repetitions on one side, switch to the other side.

TIPS

- Don't let the wrist curl in or the shoulder of the working arm roll forward when pulling the handle in.
- Start far enough away from the pulley machine so that you create tension on the cable when the arm is fully extended.

Variation: Tall-Kneeling Single-Arm Band Pull-In

Perform the tall-kneeling single-arm band pull-in with a long resistance band wrapped around a bar.

SEATED ROW

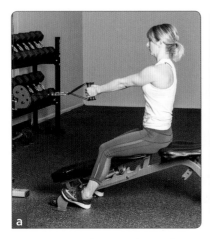 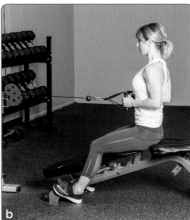

Figure 8.58 Seated row: *(a)* starting position; *(b)* row.

MUSCLES

Primary: lats, midtraps, rhomboids

Secondary: biceps, rear delts

MOVEMENT

1. Sit on the seat with the feet placed firmly against the foot supports. Grasp a V-handle attached to the cable machine at chest height with both hands.
2. Keeping the spine in neutral, row the handle in toward the upper belly, keeping the elbows tucked.
3. Return the handle to the starting position in a controlled manner.

TIPS

- Minimal movement should occur in the spine during this exercise. Don't let the upper back round and don't lean back excessively.
- Don't let the shoulders roll forward during the rowing portion of the movement. Keep the chest up and squeeze the shoulder blades together.

CHEST-SUPPORTED DUMBBELL ROW

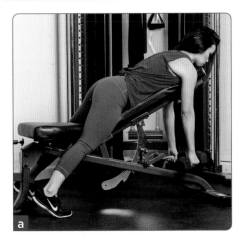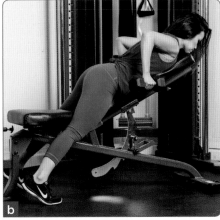

Figure 8.59 Chest-supported dumbbell row: *(a)* starting position; *(b)* row.

MUSCLES

Primary: lats, midtraps, rhomboids

Secondary: biceps, rear delts

MOVEMENT

1. Holding a dumbbell in each hand, lie prone across an incline bench with the feet planted firmly on the floor. Position the chin just on top of the bench.
2. Pull the dumbbells in toward the torso, keeping the elbows tucked and the forearms roughly vertical relative to the ground.
3. Squeeze the shoulder blades together at the top of the movement and then return the dumbbells to the starting position in a controlled manner.

TIPS

- Don't let the shoulders roll forward during the rowing portion of the movement. Keep the chest up and squeeze the shoulder blades together.
- Don't rely on momentum to row the dumbbells. Use strict form and control the weights at every portion of the movement.

LANDMINE ROW

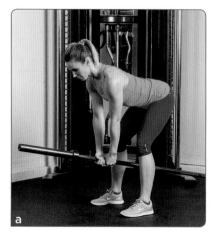 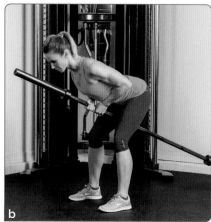

Figure 8.60 Landmine row: *(a)* starting position; *(b)* row.

MUSCLES

Primary: lats, midtraps, rhomboids

Secondary: biceps, rear delts, erector spinae

MOVEMENT

1. Place a barbell in a landmine position by wrapping a towel around one end and wedging it into a corner. Alternatively, you can position a barbell into a landmine device as shown.
2. Straddle the top end of the barbell, facing away from the end in the corner, and bend over at the hips with the spine in neutral and the knees slightly bent. The torso should be at approximately a 45-degree angle.
3. Grasping the top end of the barbell with both hands, pull the barbell in toward the body. Think of pulling the elbows toward the hips.
4. Squeeze the shoulder blades together at the top of the movement and then return the barbell to the starting position in a controlled manner.

TIPS

- The body position should mimic that of the Romanian deadlift. Keep the chest up and the back flat throughout the entire movement.
- Keep the body language to a minimum. The body should stay relatively still throughout the movement with just the arm working.
- When adding load, use smaller plates to prevent the weights from getting in the way of movement execution.

SINGLE-ARM ROW

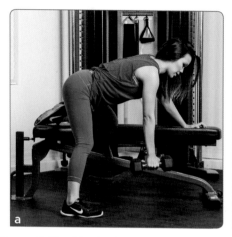 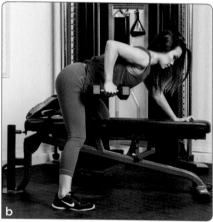

Figure 8.61 Single-arm row: *(a)* starting position; *(b)* row.

MUSCLES

Primary: lats, midtraps, rhomboids

Secondary: biceps, rear delts, erector spinae

MOVEMENT

1. Holding a dumbbell in one hand, place the opposite knee and hand on top of a bench. Plant the foot of the working side firmly on the ground.
2. While keeping the spine and the head in neutral, row the dumbbell in toward the body. The elbow should stay relatively tucked.
3. Return the dumbbell to the starting position in a controlled manner.
4. After completing all repetitions on one side, switch to the other side.

TIPS

- The foot on the ground should not be too close to the bench. Assume a wide, athletic stance to establish a good base of support.
- Keep the body language to a minimum. The body should stay relatively still throughout the movement with just the working arm in motion.
- Don't let the torso twist as you perform your repetitions.

BARBELL BENT-OVER ROW

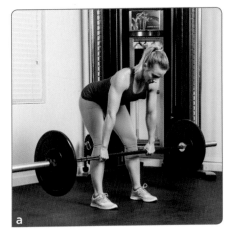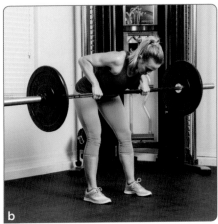

Figure 8.62   Barbell bent-over row: *(a)* starting position; *(b)* row.

MUSCLES

Primary: lats, midtraps, rhomboids

Secondary: biceps, rear delts, erector spinae

MOVEMENT

1. Assuming an overhand grip on a barbell with the hands approximately shoulder-width apart, bend over at the hips with the spine in neutral and the knees slightly bent.
2. Keeping the chest up, the shins vertical, and the torso at an approximately a 45-degree angle, pull the barbell in toward the upper belly. Think of pulling the elbows toward the hips.
3. Touch the barbell to the upper body, squeeze the shoulder blades together at the top of the movement, and then return the barbell to the starting position in a controlled manner.

TIPS

- Don't let the torso become more upright as you perform each repetition.
- Keep the body language to a minimum. The body should stay still throughout the movement with just the arms working.

Variation: Dumbbell Bent-Over Row

Perform the bent-over row with a dumbbell held in each hand.

BENT-LEG INVERTED ROW

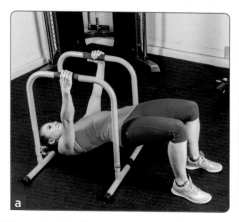 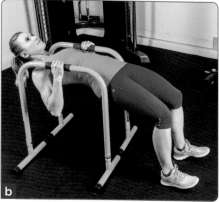

Figure 8.63 Bent-leg inverted row: *(a)* starting position; *(b)* row.

MUSCLES

Primary: lats, midtraps, rhomboids

Secondary: biceps, rear delts

MOVEMENT

1. Position an apparatus such as the Lebert Equalizer at approximately waist height.
2. From a seated position on the floor, grab the handles of the apparatus slightly wider than shoulder-width apart with the feet out in front of the body. The knees should be bent at approximately a 45-degree angle.
3. Keeping the chest up and the chin tucked, pull the torso toward the apparatus by flexing at the elbows and retracting the shoulder blades.
4. Lower the torso to the starting position in a controlled manner.

TIPS

- The more vertical your torso is to the ground, the easier the movement will be. Adjust your torso angle accordingly.
- Don't let the hips drop during the movement or as you perform more repetitions. Squeeze the glutes to maintain tension throughout the entire body.
- You may perform this movement with an overhand (pronated) grip, an underhand (supinated) grip, or a neutral grip on the bar. Use the grip variation that feels best for you.

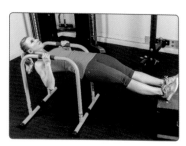

Variation: Feet-Elevated Inverted Row

Perform the inverted row with the feet elevated on a box or a bench (figure 8.64). You may use a neutral, overhand (pronated), or underhand (supinated) grip.

Figure 8.64 Feet-elevated inverted row.

SINGLE-JOINT EXERCISES

Single-joint exercises round out an already sound training program. If compound movements are the big rocks, single-joint exercises are the small pebbles that fill your training jar.

Although you can see solid physique changes by focusing on nothing but the main lifts, single-joint exercises are useful when you want to target certain body parts. These exercises can help improve weak links in physique and strength and should not be considered inferior to other movements.

Generally, you should add these exercises to a workout after you have performed the compound exercises. Single-joint exercises can be done for a greater number of repetitions using lighter weight.

This section includes just a sampling of single-joint exercises from which to choose. My clients tend to enjoy and tolerate these movements. Of course, many single-joint exercises are not mentioned, and you are encouraged to perform them at your discretion according to your goals.

DUMBBELL LATERAL RAISE

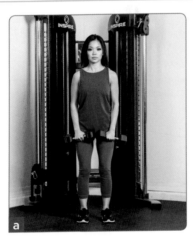 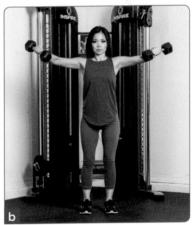

Figure 8.65 Dumbbell lateral raise: *(a)* starting position; *(b)* raise.

MUSCLES
Primary: lateral delts

MOVEMENT
1. Stand and hold a dumbbell in each hand.
2. Raise the dumbbells out to the sides with the palms facing the ground and a soft bend in the elbows.
3. When the elbows are level with the chin and the forearms are approximately parallel to the ground, lower the dumbbells to the starting position in a controlled manner.

- Avoid excessive body language when performing this exercise. You should be using the delts to raise the dumbbells rather than momentum from the hips.
- Imagine pouring a pitcher of water at the top of the movement. The pinkies should be higher than the thumbs and the elbows should be up nice and high.
- You don't need much load to feel this movement working. Rather than focusing on lifting heavier weight with this exercise, focus on activating the lateral delts.

DUMBBELL UPRIGHT ROW

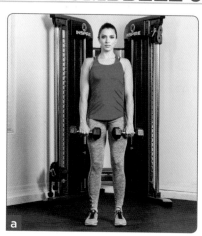 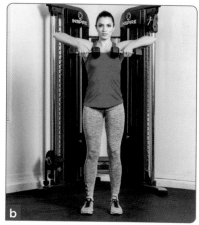

Figure 8.66   Dumbbell upright row: *(a)* starting position; *(b)* row.

MUSCLES

Primary: lateral delts, traps

Secondary: biceps

MOVEMENT

1. Stand and hold a dumbbell in each hand, palms facing and resting on the thighs. Have a slight bend in the elbows.
2. Pull the dumbbells up to just below the chin, keeping them close to the body and leading with the elbows.
3. Lower the dumbbells to the starting position in a controlled manner.

TIPS

- Always keep the elbows higher than the hands.
- Don't jerk or swing the body when performing this movement. The torso should stay relatively still, and only the arms should move.
- Err on the side of using lighter dumbbells instead of heavier weights to prevent shoulder injury.

Variation 1: Band Upright Row

Perform the upright row with a long resistance band. The band should be looped under the heels with the feet positioned approximately shoulder-width apart.

Variation 2: Cable Upright Row

Perform the upright row using the handle attachment of a pulley machine. The handle should be attached to the lowest possible position.

DUMBBELL FRONT RAISE

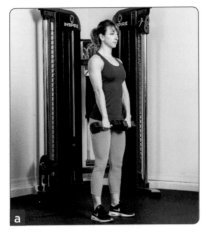 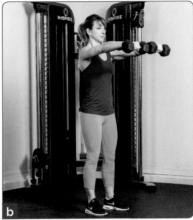

Figure 8.67 Dumbbell front raise: *(a)* starting position; *(b)* raise.

MUSCLES

Primary: anterior delts

MOVEMENT

1. Stand and hold a dumbbell in each hand in front of the body with the palms facing the thighs.
2. Raise the dumbbells out in front of the body with the palms facing the ground and a soft bend in the elbows.
3. Reverse the motion when the elbows are level with the chin. The forearms should be approximately parallel to the ground.
4. Lower the dumbbells to the starting position in a controlled manner.

TIPS

- Avoid excessive body language when performing this exercise. You should be using the delts to raise the dumbbells rather than momentum from the hips.
- You don't need much load to feel this movement working. Rather than focusing on lifting heavier weight with this exercise, focus on activating the front delts.

PRONE REAR DELT RAISE

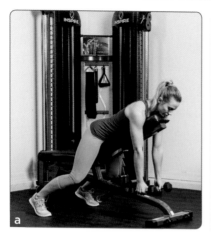 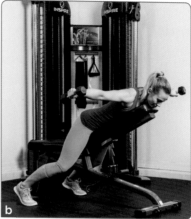

Figure 8.68 Prone rear delt raise: *(a)* starting position; *(b)* raise.

MUSCLES

Primary: rear delts

MOVEMENT

1. Hold a dumbbell in each hand. Lie prone across an incline bench with the feet planted firmly on the floor. Position the chin just on top of the bench.
2. Raise the dumbbells out to each side with the palms facing the ground and a soft bend in the elbows.
3. Form a T with the torso and the arms at the top of the movement.
4. Lower the dumbbells to the starting position.

TIP

You don't need much load to feel this movement working. Rather than focusing on lifting heavier weight with this exercise, focus on activating the rear delts.

SINGLE-ARM CABLE REAR DELT RAISE

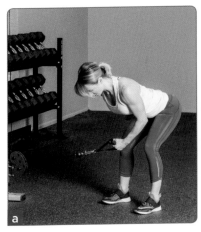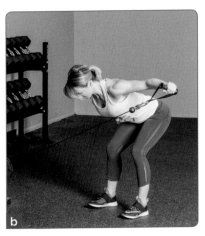

Figure 8.69 Single-arm cable rear delt raise: *(a)* starting position; *(b)* raise.

MUSCLES
Primary: rear delts

MOVEMENT
1. Attach a handle attachment to the lowest position on a cable machine. Stand beside the machine with the feet approximately shoulder-width apart and the knees slightly bent. With the outside hand, grasp the handle, palm up. Pull to remove any slack from the pulley.
2. Keeping the back flat and the head neutral, straighten the working arm to the side. Power should come from the rear delt. Pull until the forearm is approximately parallel to the ground. Keep the wrist of the working hand in neutral position.
3. Return to the starting position in a controlled manner.
4. After finishing all repetitions on one side, switch to the other side and repeat.

TIPS
- Remember that this exercise targets the rear delt.
- Don't use momentum to pull the handle back.
- Use a light enough weight that you can feel the rear delt working.

INCLINE DUMBBELL FLY

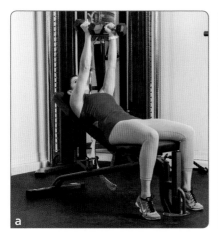 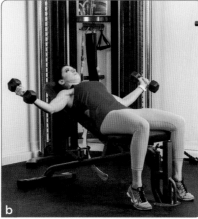

Figure 8.70 Incline dumbbell fly: *(a)* starting position; *(b)* action.

MUSCLES

Primary: pecs

MOVEMENT

1. Hold a dumbbell in each hand. Sit on an incline bench positioned at approximately a 30- to 45-degree angle.
2. Extend the arms above the body and turn the palms toward each other.
3. With a slight bend in the elbows, lower the arms to the sides in a controlled manner until the palms face the ceiling.
4. Reverse the motion and bring the arms back above the body.
5. Repeat.

TIPS

- Be careful not to cut the range of motion short as you perform more repetitions and become fatigued. If this starts to happen, end the set early or grab a lighter pair of dumbbells.
- At the bottom of the movement, make sure you feel a stretch in the pecs.

CABLE CROSSOVER

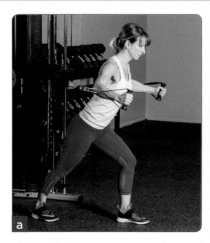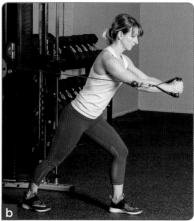

Figure 8.71 Cable crossover: *(a)* starting position; *(b)* press.

MUSCLES

Primary: pecs

MOVEMENT

1. Attach two handle attachments to a crossover cable machine, each at approximately midheight and even with each other. Stand with your back to the machine and grip a handle in each hand, palms turned toward each other and elbows just below shoulder height and bent. Assume a lunge position.
2. Keeping the back straight and the neck neutral, press the handles forward and together, keeping the palms facing each other.
3. Return the handles to the starting position in a controlled manner. You should feel a slight stretch across the pecs.
4. For the next set, switch legs so that the other leg is in front.

TIP

Maintain a slight bend in the elbows throughout the execution of the movement.

STRAIGHT-ARM PULLDOWN

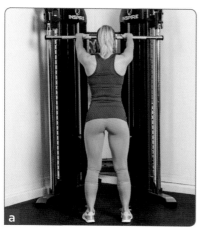 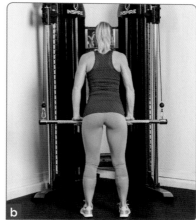

Figure 8.72   Straight-arm pulldown: *(a)* starting position; *(b)* action.

MUSCLES

Primary: lats

Secondary: triceps

MOVEMENT

1. Stand and grasp a wide bar from the top pulley of a cable machine with the hands slightly wider than shoulder-width apart and the palms facing down. Take one step back. The arms should be fully extended with a slight bend in the elbows.
2. Pull the bar down while keeping the arms straight by contracting the lats until the hands touch the thighs.
3. Return the bar to the starting position in a controlled manner.

TIPS

- The hips should be bent at a slight 15- to 30-degree angle. If necessary, take an extra step back from the cable machine to achieve the correct starting position.
- You can also perform this movement on a lat pulldown machine.

DUMBBELL PULLOVER

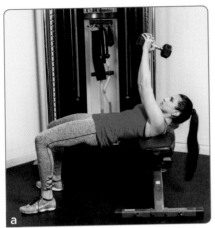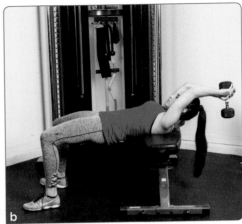

Figure 8.73 Dumbbell pullover: *(a)* starting position; *(b)* action.

MUSCLES

Primary: pectorals

Secondary: deltoids, lats, triceps, gluteals

MOVEMENT

1. Lie perpendicular on a bench with the shoulders resting on the bench. The feet should be on the floor approximately shoulder-width apart, and knees should be at approximately a 90-degree angle.
2. Grasp a dumbbell vertically in both hands and hold it above the chest. The arms should be fully extended with a slight bend in the elbows.
3. Slowly lower the dumbbell behind the head following an arc path.
4. Return the dumbbell to the starting position in a controlled manner.

TIPS

- Although this is primarily an upper-body exercise, you'll notice that the body position is not unlike that of the hip thrust. Work the lower body as well by squeezing the glutes while performing your repetitions.
- The hands should hold onto the underside of the dumbbell head.
- Let the dumbbell go back only as far as comfortable. You should feel a stretch in the pecs when performing this exercise.

FACE PULL

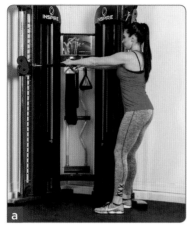 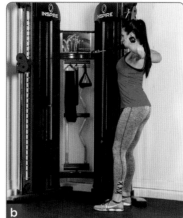

Figure 8.74   Face pull: *(a)* starting position; *(b)* action.

MUSCLES

Primary: rear delts

Secondary: rhomboids

MOVEMENT

1. Stand and grasp the handles of a rope attached to a cable machine at approximately chest height. The feet should be approximately shoulder-width apart, and the arms should be fully extended.
2. Pull the rope toward the face while separating the hands and keeping the elbows high.
3. Return the rope to the starting position in a controlled manner.

TIPS

- Don't shrug the shoulders while performing this movement.
- Think of pulling the rope apart as it moves toward you rather than simply pulling back.
- You may prefer to use a staggered stance with one foot forward, especially as you increase the load.

Variation: Band Face Pull

Perform the face pull using a long resistance band wrapped around a power rack or an equally sturdy apparatus.

ROPE TRICEPS EXTENSION

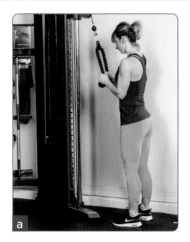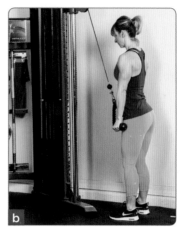

Figure 8.75 Rope triceps extension: *(a)* starting position; *(b)* triceps extension.

MUSCLES
Primary: triceps

MOVEMENT
1. Grasp a rope attached to the top of a cable machine with both hands.
2. Press the arms down, keeping the elbows close to the sides. Contract the triceps.
3. Reverse the motion to return to the starting position.

TIPS
- You may prefer to use a staggered stance with one foot forward, especially as you increase the load.
- When using the rope, you can also pull the rope apart as you extend the elbows.

DUMBBELL SKULL CRUSHER

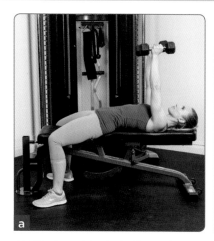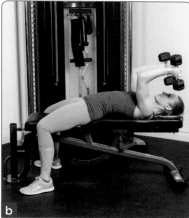

Figure 8.76 Dumbbell skull crusher: *(a)* starting position; *(b)* action.

MUSCLES

Primary: triceps

MOVEMENT

1. Hold a dumbbell in each hand. Lie back on a bench with the arms fully extended and perpendicular to the floor. Plant the feet firmly on the floor.
2. Slowly lower the dumbbells by flexing the elbows until the dumbbells are close to your head.
3. Reverse the motion by extending the elbows.

TIPS

- Contrary to what the name implies, the dumbbells should not crush—or even touch—your skull. Be sure to lower the dumbbells in a controlled manner to avoid dropping the weights on your head and causing injury.
- Keep the upper arms stationary throughout the duration of the movement.

DUMBBELL CURL

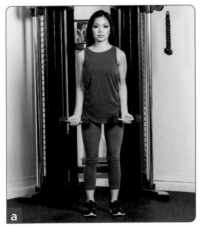 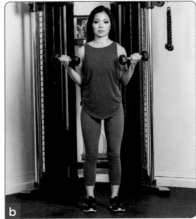

Figure 8.77 Dumbbell curl: *(a)* starting position; *(b)* curl.

MUSCLES

Primary: biceps

MOVEMENT

1. Stand and hold a dumbbell in each hand, arms fully extended at the sides of the body. The palms should face forward.
2. Flex the elbows and raise the dumbbells while keeping the upper arms stationary until the dumbbells are at shoulder level.
3. Squeeze the biceps and then slowly lower the dumbbells to the starting position.

TIPS

- Be careful not to swing the weights up by using excessive momentum of the body. The torso should remain relatively still.
- Offset the dumbbell by holding the handle on the lateral side to increase biceps activation.

HAMMER CURL

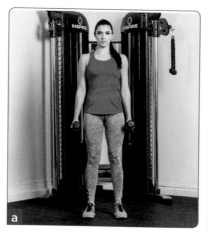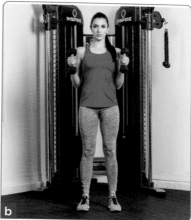

Figure 8.78 Hammer curl: *(a)* starting position; *(b)* curl.

MUSCLES

Primary: biceps

MOVEMENT

1. Stand and hold a dumbbell in each hand, arms fully extended at the sides of the body. The palms should face each other.
2. Flex the elbows and raise the dumbbells while keeping the upper arms stationary until the dumbbells are at shoulder level.
3. Squeeze the biceps and then slowly lower the dumbbells to the starting position.

TIPS

- Be careful not to swing the weights up by using excessive momentum of the body. The torso should remain relatively still.
- Holding the dumbbells toward the top of the handles can lead to a smoother, more fluid motion.

POSTERIOR PELVIC TILT PLANK

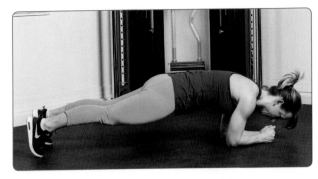

Figure 8.79   Posterior pelvic tilt plank.

MUSCLES
Primary: rectus abdominis, internal obliques, external obliques, gluteals

MOVEMENT
1. Assume a plank position on the forearms with the elbows directly beneath the shoulders and the feet slightly narrower than shoulder-width apart.
2. Squeezing the hands into fists, pull the feet and elbows toward each other while squeezing the glutes, pressing the thighs together, and squeezing the quads.
3. Hold for time.

TIPS
- The first few times you do this, you may not be able to last long until your entire body starts shaking like a leaf. This outcome is normal, but over time your strength endurance will improve.
- Keep a very slight bend in the knees and round the upper back to allow more posterior pelvic tilt.
- Make sure you contract the glutes as hard as possible during this exercise.

HOLLOW BODY HOLD

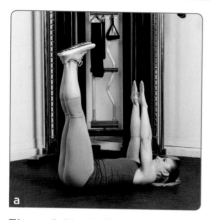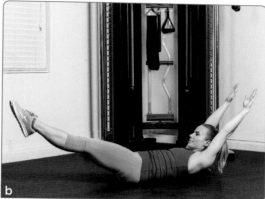

Figure 8.80 Hollow body hold: (a) starting position; (b) hold.

MUSCLES

Primary: rectus abdominis, internal obliques, external obliques

MOVEMENT

1. Lie in a supine position with the arms straight and held in front and legs in the air. Flatten the lumbar spine so that the low back is touching the floor.
2. Slowly lower the arms back and legs down in front of the body while keeping the lumbar spine in contact with the floor. Find the lowest position at which you can hold the arms and legs straight without actually touching the floor.
3. Hold for time.

TIPS

- The first few times you do this, you'll likely have to hold the arms and legs higher above the floor. Over time, as you increase strength endurance, you'll be able to lower the arms and legs.
- Think of pulling the belly button toward the floor while performing this movement.

SIDE PLANK

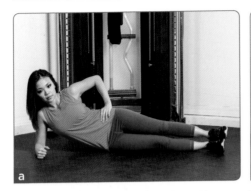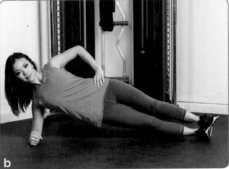

Figure 8.81 Side plank: *(a)* starting position; *(b)* plank.

MUSCLES

Primary: obliques

MOVEMENT

1. Lie on your side on the ground with the elbow directly beneath the shoulder and the feet stacked on top of each another.
2. Prop up the torso on the resting elbow and then raise the hips off the ground so that the body forms a straight line from head to toe.
3. Hold for time. Repeat on the other side.

TIPS

- Many people like to put the free arm on the hip, but you can also lay it flat against the side of the body or hold it straight up.
- To progress this movement, raise and hold the top leg in the air.

CABLE PALLOF PRESS

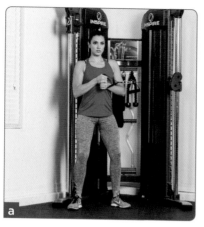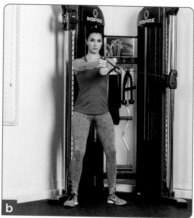

Figure 8.82 Cable Pallof press: *(a)* starting position; *(b)* press.

MUSCLES

Primary: obliques

Secondary: gluteals

MOVEMENT

1. Position a standard pulley handle to a cable machine at approximately chest height. Grab the handle with both hands and stand perpendicular to the pulley handle on the machine with the feet just outside shoulder-width apart. The body should be far enough away from the machine that the cable is under tension.
2. Beginning with the hands at the chest and a slight bend in the knees, squeeze the glutes and then press the cable away from the torso, fully extending the arms.
3. Return the hands to the starting position in a controlled manner.
4. After completing all repetitions on one side, switch sides.

TIPS

- This movement should be slow and controlled. Rather than trying to complete the repetitions as quickly as possible, focus on engaging the core and keeping the body tight.
- The cable is going to want to rotate your body inward, so make sure to keep tension in the body. Only the arms should move, not the torso or hips.
- If you find it difficult to prevent the hips from moving, try widening your stance or lightening the load.

Variation: Band Pallof Press

Perform the band Pallof press with a long resistance band wrapped around a power rack or a similarly sturdy implement at approximately chest height.

LEG EXTENSION

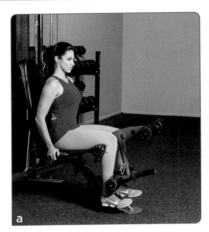 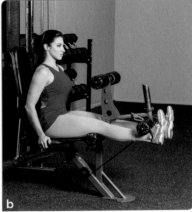

Figure 8.83   Leg extension: *(a)* starting position; *(b)* leg extension.

MUSCLES

Primary: quadriceps

MOVEMENT

1. Sit on a leg extension machine with the feet hooked under the pads and the hands grasping the side bars. Adjust the pads so that the knees rest at approximately a 90-degree angle.
2. Extend the knees while keeping the rest of the body stationary.
3. Lower the weight to the starting position in a controlled manner.

TIPS

- Don't rely on momentum to lift the weight.
- Adjust the machine so that you can achieve a full range of motion rather than do partial repetitions.

STABILITY BALL LEG CURL

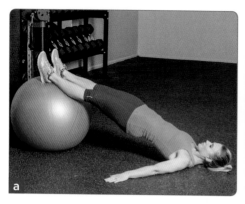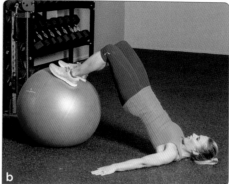

Figure 8.84 Stability ball leg curl: *(a)* starting position; *(b)* leg curl.

MUSCLES

Primary: hamstrings, gluteals

MOVEMENT

1. Lie in a supine position with the legs fully extended and the ankles and calves resting on a stability ball.
2. With the hands on the ground palms down, extend the hips and squeeze the glutes so that the body forms a straight line from shoulders to toes.
3. Flex the knees and curl the stability ball into the body while keeping the hips off the ground.
4. Extend the knees and return the stability ball to the starting position in a controlled manner.

TIPS

- Don't let the hips drop as you perform the repetitions.
- As you tire, be careful not to increase the speed of the repetitions. Keep the movements slow and controlled, especially as you move the stability ball away from the body.

LYING LEG CURL

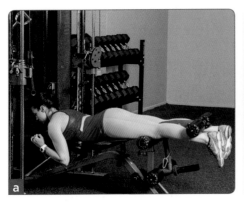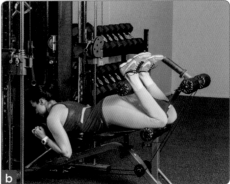

Figure 8.85 Lying leg curl: *(a)* starting position; *(b)* leg curl.

MUSCLES

Primary: hamstrings

MOVEMENT

1. Lie face down (prone) on a lying leg curl machine with the pad of the lever against the back of the ankles. Grab the handles of the machine.
2. Curl the legs by flexing the knees while keeping the torso lying flat against the pad.
3. After fully contracting the hamstrings, lower the weight to the starting position in a controlled manner.

TIP

If possible, use a lying leg curl machine that has an angled pad as opposed to a flat pad to create greater hamstring recruitment.

NORDIC HAMSTRING CURL

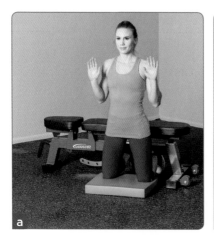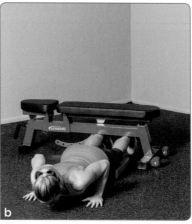

Figure 8.86 Nordic hamstring curl: *(a)* starting position; *(b)* hamstring curl.

MUSCLES

Primary: hamstrings

MOVEMENT

1. From a tall-kneeling position, place a pad under the knees and hook the feet under a sturdy implement.
2. While squeezing the glutes, lower the torso to the ground in a controlled manner without allowing the hips to flex. The eccentric phase should take three to five seconds.
3. Catch the body on the ground with the hands and then lightly push the torso back up to the starting position.

TIPS

- Many people make the mistake of folding over at the hips when lowering the body to the ground rather than keeping the body straight. Having a faster eccentric phase at first is preferable to allowing the hips to shoot back.
- Control the eccentric phase as much as possible. At first, you may feel as though you're simply flopping to the ground because of insufficient hamstring strength, but you will improve over time.

DUMBBELL SINGLE-LEG STANDING CALF RAISE

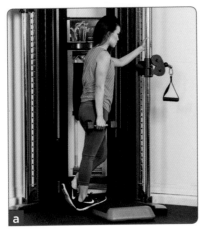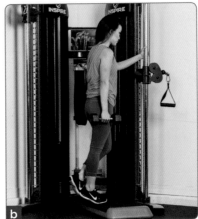

Figure 8.87 Dumbbell single-leg standing calf raise: *(a)* starting position; *(b)* calf raise.

MUSCLES

Primary: gastrocnemius, soleus

MOVEMENT

1. Holding a dumbbell in one hand, place the front half of the foot of the same side on a flat, sturdy platform. The arch and the heel of the working leg should extend off the platform, and the other hand should hold onto a support for balance.
2. With a slight bend in the knee of the working leg, lift the heel by extending the ankle until the calf is fully contracted.
3. Slowly lower the heel to the starting position in a controlled manner.
4. After completing repetitions on one side, switch to the other side.

TIP

The foot of the nonworking leg can be wrapped around the ankle of the working leg or bent back off the platform.

CALF PRESS

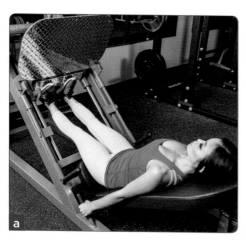 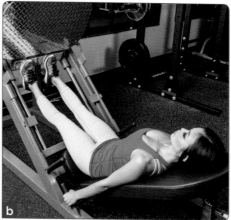

Figure 8.88 Calf press: *(a)* starting position; *(b)* press.

MUSCLES

Primary: calves

MOVEMENT

1. Sit on the seat of a leg press machine and adjust the distance of the platform so that the feet can reach the platform when the legs are fully extended. Position the toes and balls of the feet on the bottom of the platform at approximately shoulder-width apart with the heels extending off.
2. With the torso leaning against the back padding, push the platform away by extending the ankles until the calves are fully contracted.
3. Slowly lower the heels to the starting position in a controlled manner.

TIPS

- Slow the eccentric portion up to a count of 10 to get the most out of the movement.
- Adjust the seat position so that the calves are fully stretched at the bottom of the movement.

ACTIONABLE ITEMS

Chapter 8 shows you how to execute all the exercises you'll need for my training programs. By mastering these movements, you'll be able to build strength, pack on muscle, transform your physique, and change your life. As you practice these movements, I encourage you to pay attention to every repetition you perform so that they become second nature to you. You can then progress to setting personal records in the gym and reaching your strength and performance goals. You're on your way to becoming a whole new you!

CHAPTER 9

Cardio and Glute Circuits

In 2004 I was a high school freshman. Like any budding teenager, I was growing into my identity and trying to figure out who I was. I clung desperately to the opinions of others and fruitlessly tried to conform to the ideals that others deemed desirable: thin, hardworking, smart, athletic, fun to be around—the whole package.

I was a dedicated student. It made sense to me: show up, do the work, study the materials, and get the grade. So when it came to keeping my figure trim, I reasoned that the approach was the same: show up, burn the calories through whatever means possible, and the body would mold itself into a svelte figure with slim hips and a flat abdomen.

It started innocently enough. I was on the varsity cross country team as well as the varsity swim team, so I ran with my teammates in the afternoon, went home for a quick snack, and then scurried off to two hours of swim practice. *Wow*, my peers gasped, *look at you go!* I was the object of admiration, and I reveled in it.

THE DREADED C WORD: CARDIO

Of course, I took great pride in the fact that I did more cardio than any of my classmates did. I slowly started to shed body fat over time, and when I noticed this happening—and especially when others started commenting on the changes, applauding just how attractive I was becoming—I was hooked.

Rather than train for performance, I started exercising for the sole purpose of losing weight. Forget bringing down my 5K time—I had more important matters to tend to!

Eventually, my weekend downtime faded away as I started waking up early to sneak off to the gym. I'd plug in my earphones and pedal away on the stationary bike for hours, willing the time to go by faster. Or I'd go out for a 10-mile (16 km) run, hating every step I took. I'd then shuffle back home, exhausted, and step on the scale in hopes that I'd lost weight and become more attractive in my peers' eyes.

I had become the cardio queen within a matter of months. And I hated every bit of it. I'd grown to despise cardio, or any form of exercise for that matter. What had previously been a source of stress relief and excitement had turned into a form of punishment. I didn't allow myself to enjoy my day until I had completed my self-mandated cardio. I convinced myself that I would gain body fat overnight if I ever happened to miss a day on the treadmill.

The saddest part about all this is that my physique slimmed down only marginally and only for a little while. After a few months, I started gaining weight as my caloric consumption increased because I overestimated my energy expenditure during exercise. In a panic, I would log more minutes on the bike, which would then make me hungrier, which would make me overeat, and I'd gain even more weight. I was stuck in a vicious cycle, and I was starting to believe that I was never destined to look lean and muscular.

Perhaps my story hits a little too close to home for you. Maybe you're living this right now. The good news, now that you're in possession of this book, is that you're in good hands. I used to think that there wasn't a light at the end of the tunnel, that I was doomed to spend the rest of my life hating exercise and counting down the minutes until my workout was done for the day. I couldn't fathom there being any other way.

Resistance training saved the day, and I won't be surprised if it ends up being a godsend for you, too. Although I once believed that not exercising to the point of exhaustion would lead to immediate physique sabotage, I now understand that it's not always about exercising more, but about exercising smarter.

I'm not here to demonize cardio. Rather, the purpose of this chapter is to explore cardio as it relates to the big picture. When is it appropriate to perform cardio, and if it is, at what doses? How can you fit cardio into your program so that it can help, not hinder, your progress toward your goals?

REASONS TO MINIMIZE CARDIO

Cardio has a place in a well-designed program for some people, depending on goals and a person's unique lifestyle factors. But the thinking that more is always better is misguided and can get you into a lot of trouble.

I've always loved what my friend and mentor Layne Norton says about cardio: "Cardio should be like a girl's skirt: long enough to cover the subject, but short enough to keep things interesting."

Sauciness aside, when training for aesthetic purposes or when chasing strength gains in the gym, cardio should be kept to a minimum. For most clients, in fact, I prescribe zero formal cardio to begin with and let proper nutrition create most of the caloric deficit.

Most people tend to think that the more calories you burn and the fewer calories you ingest, the faster and better the fat-loss results will be, but what these people fail to consider is that these drastic measures are not sustainable. Yes, you may be able to keep up an extreme regimen for a few weeks, but at what cost? What sacrifices will you have to make in your life to make this happen, and are you willing to continue doing this indefinitely? I'm usually met with a blank stare when I ask these questions.

Think of it this way: The more cardio you do on a regular basis, the more you're going to have to add to continue seeing physique results. For that reason, I recommend taking the minimum effective dose route. The ultimate goal, after all, is to minimize suffering and maximize enjoyment so that you can adhere to the program.

For most women, a tremendous amount of physique progress can be made without any formal cardio. A solid regimen of proper nutrition (keeping overall calories in check and keeping protein intake high) and resistance training should be enough to do the trick for the vast majority. Only if progress stalls do I consider sprinkling in some cardio, although I'll often opt instead to manipulate a client's nutrition program. We have only so much time in the day, after all, and we're all busy.

Here's my rationale: The calorie expenditure that occurs as a result of cardiovascular exercise is actually quite low—surprisingly low. I once mistakenly believed that an hour of trudging away on the treadmill torched 2,000 calories (because, you know, that's what the treadmill told me), and I took that as license to overindulge after my workout. The truth is that jogging for an hour at a steady pace of 9 minutes per mile (5 min, 35 sec per km) probably burned only 300 to 350 calories.

I don't know about you, but I'm a busy gal, and I have many other things that I would rather get done in that amount of time. Moreover, I can save myself both time and money (on food, that is) by simply shaving a few hundred calories off my daily diet. The choice is a no-brainer to me.

Of course, if you're the type of person who prefers to eat more food and perform more cardio, feel free to do so. But be careful not to overdo it, because you don't want your cardio to have a negative effect on your strength training. Remember that strength training takes priority.

ISN'T THAT NEAT?

We should also consider the role that nonexercise activity thermogenesis, or NEAT, plays in caloric expenditure. NEAT is essentially any physical activity performed throughout the day that is not formal exercise. These activities include fidgeting, adjusting your posture, and even typing on your laptop.

NEAT makes up a surprisingly large proportion of your daily energy expenditure, and it can burn far more calories throughout the day than a formal workout does (Livingstone et al. 1991). In sedentary people, NEAT may make up as little as 15 percent of daily energy expenditure, but it can go as high as 32 percent or more in active people.

A number of factors influence NEAT, including occupation (do you work a desk job, or are you on your feet all day?), your environmental surroundings, and the weather. A genetic component applies as well.

Take, for instance, my friend, whom we'll call Jean. Jean is a wife and a mother of two, and she keeps herself busy all day tending to her family. Her husband reports that from the moment she wakes up to the moment she goes to bed at night, she never sits down. This account may be a slight exaggeration, but the point is that she is constantly on her feet, always bustling about. In large part because of her high daily NEAT, she rocks a slim figure year round. She doesn't spend that much time in the gym. She's healthy from head to toe, and she has absolutely no need to add formal cardio to her exercise regimen.

Additionally, the more formal exercise you perform, the more your NEAT can drop. Put another way, doing too much in the way of working out can leave you exhausted, leading you to become less active outside the gym overall. This typically happens to people without them realizing it. So if you end up doing so much in the gym that you don't do enough outside the gym, doesn't that defeat the whole purpose?

If you're an endurance athlete or if your primary goal is to become a better runner, then of course you would want to make running your primary form of exercise. In that case, you'd be training for a specific purpose, and prioritizing running would lead to the best improvement in performance. But chances are that's not you, and you're here because you want to get stronger and improve your body composition without tormenting yourself in the process.

CARDIO AND HEART HEALTH

Ah, but you may be wondering how I could possibly be telling people *not* to jog multiple days per week when cardio work is crucial for heart health. Isn't that recommendation irresponsible of me as a fitness coach?

The truth is that resistance training is just as effective at inducing cardiovascular adaptations with the added bonus of increasing lean body mass, strength, and day-to-day functioning. More specifically, both cardio and strength training improve maximal oxygen uptake and endothelial function, decrease oxidized low-density lipoprotein levels, and increase calcium transport in the skeletal muscle. Strength training additionally improves antioxidant status (Schjerve et al. 2008).

And let's not forget high-intensity interval training (HIIT). In this form of aerobic training, low-intensity exercise is interspersed with high-intensity bursts of effort. HIIT can be helpful in increasing whole-body and skeletal muscle capacity to oxidize carbohydrate and fat (Perry et al. 2008). This goal can be accomplished with just 15 minutes of intense exercise spread out over a two-week period (Gibala and McGee 2008), an alarmingly small volume of training. In addition, research shows that HIIT tends to be superior to steady-state cardio for fat loss (Tremblay, Simoneau, and Bouchard 1994; Trapp et al. 2008), leading to increased loss of subcutaneous fat. In addition, a study on rats showed that high-intensity exercise can suppress appetite (Bilski et al. 2009). Finally, HIIT has greater excess post-exercise oxygen consumption (EPOC), which means that high-intensity exercise, although shorter in duration, burns more calories in the hours following the workout than does lower-intensity exercise such as low-intensity steady-state cardio, or LISS (Laforgia, Withers, and Gore 2006).

This news is great for those of you who begrudgingly pedal away on the stationary bike for 30 minutes at a time for the sake of your health. Those days are long over for me, and it's a relief to see that I didn't shoot myself in the foot by handing in my cardio queen card. If you're anything like me and you're easily bored by performing the same repetitive motion over and over, then you should be just fine adhering primarily to a resistance-training regimen.

All of this to say that, for many reasons, if you're going to perform cardio, then the high-intensity kind might be the option to go for. But each method has pros and cons, which I'll go over in the next section.

USING CARDIO

Now that we've discussed what cardio—both the steady-state kind and the high-intensity kind—does for your body, how can we apply it (if at all) to a sound exercise regimen? I'm not here to give you a one-size-fits-all program, so what's optimal for you won't necessarily be what's best for your training partner.

Here are some variables to consider if you should incorporate cardio in your regimen:

- Your current fitness goal
- The types of cardio modalities you enjoy, if any
- The time you have to devote to working out
- Existing injuries
- General day-to-day energy

If in doubt, err on the side of doing less. No, that's not a typo. Many women make the mistake of doing far too much cardio, thinking that they're the exception to the rule. I'm sorry to say that you are probably not the exception.

You should use cardio only when you've manipulated your nutrition as much as you can and you've ruled out sleep and stress as confounding variables to your progress. Obviously, you should be gauging your progress using the appropriate measures beyond simply weighing yourself on a scale. We'll cover this concept in depth in chapter 12, so don't worry about it for now.

Let's summarize what we've covered so far: Keep cardio to a minimum for as long as possible, prioritize strength training, let your diet do most of the work, and sprinkle in cardio only on an as-needed basis. Now, if you've determined that it is indeed time to lace up your running shoes, let's figure out the logistics of going about this.

Your Questions Answered

Q: My exercise regimen for the past several years has entailed hours and hours of cardio per week. How should I wean myself off all the biking and jogging I've been doing? Should I cut it out cold turkey or slowly dwindle it down?

A: I'm alright with either approach. I guess it depends mostly on what you're comfortable with. I've had clients see great success by cutting out the six hours per week of steady-state cardio they were performing right away and replacing it with three to four hours a week of strength training. Their body composition started to improve almost immediately, and they reported instantly feeling more vibrant and energetic. Alternatively, you can cut out an hour or so per week until you've replaced it with a few days of low-intensity leisure walking (primarily for stress relief) or a small dose of moderate-intensity cardio.

Although HIIT may take up less time, it also is inherently more dangerous. Exercise forms such as sprinting include a high risk of getting hurt, which could seriously derail your progress if you're not careful. In addition, some people simply flat-out do not enjoy HIIT, and they dread the pain and discomfort that accompanies that kind of exercise. If this is the case, HIIT is probably not worth performing. On the other hand, LISS can become monotonous, especially for those who are easily bored.

Leisure walking is my cardio modality of choice, both for myself and for most of my clients. This form of LISS is my favorite form of exercise outside strength training for the following reasons:

- It relieves stress. I can unwind from the long day, take time to gather my thoughts, call a friend, listen to a podcast, or simply let my mind wander. In addition, walking helps get the blood flowing through my muscles.
- It gets me off the couch after a day of working at my desk.
- It's easy on my joints. I don't have to worry about getting shin splints or hurting my hip flexors by strolling through my neighborhood. Walking presents virtually zero risk of injury and zero crossover effect into my strength training.

The last point is the most important to me. My goal in fitness is not only to build muscle and get strong but also to feel good and stay injury-free over the long term. This priority should be yours as well.

The great thing about leisure walking is that just about anyone can do it. You don't need any special equipment, and it costs nothing.

Besides walking, you can choose from an infinite array of cardio modalities. My second favorite mode is incline walking on a treadmill (when the weather isn't cooperating or when it's too late at night to stroll alone safely). Keep in mind that cardio forms that are more concentric in nature, such as cycling, incline walking, and sled pushes, won't induce as much soreness, which means that you'll still feel good when you lift weights. Jogging and hiking downhill, however, involve a good deal of eccentric work that can negatively affect your gym performance.

Your Questions Answered

Q: I've heard that doing cardio in a fasted state burns more body fat than doing it in a fed state. Does this suggestion have any merit?

A: Within bodybuilding circles in particular, people widely believed that fasted cardio (that is, performing cardio first thing in the morning on an empty stomach) yielded superior fat-burning results (Phillips 1999). A 2014 study by Schoenfeld et al., however, has since debunked this myth. In this intervention, 20 healthy young women were assigned to either a fasted training group or a fed training group. All participants performed one hour of steady-state aerobic exercise three days per week while following a dietary plan that put each of them in a caloric deficit. Although participants in both groups lost body weight and fat mass over four weeks, the differences between the groups were not statistically significant.

The moral of the story is that if you are using cardio for fat-loss purposes, you may do so in a fasted or fed state according to personal preference. The evidence does not support the long-held belief that fasted cardio is better.

In general, if you have to do cardio, then you should choose the form that you most enjoy and that you're most likely to adhere to consistently. You can perform HIIT if you'd prefer to get it over with quickly. I would start with two sessions a week consisting of six to eight sets of 15- to 20-second high-intensity bursts followed by 80 to 100 seconds of active rest. If you prefer LISS, 20 to 30 minutes three days a week should do the trick at first. Be sure to warm up and cool down properly.

Ideally, you should perform cardio workouts on a separate day from your resistance-training sessions, but if you can't do that, then you should do them either in a separate session (for example, do cardio in the morning and lift in the evening) or immediately after your resistance-training workouts. Be sure to take at least one day, ideally two or three days, of rest per week to allow recovery.

Don't get greedy with cardio and don't go from 0 to 100 overnight. Again, cardio should be a supplementary form of exercise to induce positive changes in body composition.

CARDIO WITH A TWIST: GLUTE CIRCUITS

I learned about glute circuits from my mentor Bret Contreras, and I quickly got hooked on them. In 2015 I performed 10-minute glute circuits four days a week after each weight-training session throughout my six-week prep for my national-level bikini show. Paired with more than eight years of lifting experience at that time and a consistent calorie deficit, I stepped on stage with my best package yet and with much of my glute fullness retained.

These glute circuits were a welcome alternative to sprints on a stationary bike. They were fun and quick, and I got a mighty glute pump each time. More important, they never left me crippled, so the next day I would be fine to go about my regular activities.

I don't recommend performing these circuits week in and week out throughout the year. Treat them as you would regular cardio. Keep them in your arsenal for when you need to up the workout ante. More specifically, perform them only in the last phases of a dieting stint (the last four to six weeks) to retain glute mass.

The goal with glute circuits is not to get stronger over time or set personal records. This is not the time to be grinding out repetitions. Rather, focus on feeling your glutes working and achieving a solid pump each time. You can use the same weights and level of resistance week after week as long as you're feeling it in the right places.

Your Questions Answered

Q: I love running a few times a week because it's my "me" time. Will continuing to do this as a form of stress relief hinder my progress?

A: I have no issues with incorporating cardio into your regimen if it's something that you enjoy. As with all forms of exercise, it should add to your quality of life. Do you look forward to it? Is it one of the highlights of your day? Then by all means, go for it. Just keep in mind that doing too much at too high of an intensity can negatively affect your performance in the gym, which you don't want to happen if aesthetics or strength gain is your primary goal.

No matter what people say about the interference effect of cardio, it's obvious. If you're trying to train for a marathon and do weights at the same time, they're going to interfere with one another. Plan your cardio around strength training.

Start with 10- to 15-minute sessions of these glute circuits, two or three days per week. Most of you who end up performing any cardio at all won't need to do more than this if your other fat-loss variables (diet, sleep, stress, hydration) are squared away.

I've included five glute circuits to choose from. You'll recognize all these exercises from chapter 8.

Again, don't strive to lift as much weight as you can. For example, during barbell hip thrusts, some people don't feel their glutes if they use too much load, which defeats the whole purpose. Select a reasonable load or resistance that allows you to perform each movement with quality form and gets your glutes firing.

Table 9.1   Glute Circuit 1

Perform these four exercises in sequence for the prescribed number of repetitions. Rest for approximately two minutes at the end of each round. Perform three to five rounds.

Exercise	Sets	Repetitions	Rest	Page
1. Knee-banded barbell hip thrust	3 to 5	10 to 15	0	106
2. Bodyweight single-leg knee banded hip thrust	3 to 5	10 to 15 each leg	0	107
3. Hip- and knee-banded hip thrust	3 to 5	10 to 15	0	106
4. Knee-banded bodyweight hip thrust	3 to 5	10 to 15	120 s	106

Table 9.2   Glute Circuit 2

Perform these five exercises in sequence for the prescribed number of repetitions. Rest for approximately two minutes at the end of each round. Perform two or three rounds.

Exercise	Sets	Repetitions	Rest	Page
1. Knee-banded dumbbell goblet squat	2 or 3	15 to 20	0	80
2. Standing band hip abduction	2 or 3	15 to 20 each leg	0	115
3. Dumbbell glute bridge	2 or 3	15 to 20	0	102
4. Lateral walk	2 or 3	15 to 20 each leg	0	110
5. Knee-banded reverse hyperextension	2 or 3	15 to 20	120 s	95

Table 9.3   Glute Circuit 3

Perform these eight exercises in sequence for the prescribed number of repetitions. Rest for approximately two minutes at the end of each round. Perform two or three rounds.

Exercise	Sets	Repetitions	Rest	Page
1. Barbell hip thrust	2 or 3	15 to 20	0	105
2. Knee-banded fire hydrant	2 or 3	15 to 20 each leg	0	117
3. Dumbbell frog pump	2 or 3	15 to 20	0	108
4. Seated band hip abduction	2 or 3	15 to 20	0	114
5. Knee-banded feet-elevated glute bridge	2 or 3	15 to 20	0	104
6. Knee-banded fire hydrant	2 or 3	15 to 20 each leg	0	117
7. Bodyweight reverse lunge	2 or 3	15 to 20 each leg	0	86
8. Bodyweight side-lying hip abduction	2 or 3	15 to 20 each leg	120 s	113

Table 9.4 Glute Circuit 4

Perform the A set of three exercises in sequence for the prescribed number of repetitions. Rest for approximately one minute between rounds. Then move to the B set and perform each exercise for the prescribed number of repetitions. Rest for approximately one minute between rounds.

Exercise	Sets	Repetitions	Rest	Page
A1. Bodyweight back extension	2 to 4	20 to 30	0	93
A2. Seated band hip abduction	2 to 4	20 to 30	0	114
A3. Bodyweight hip thrust	2 to 4	10 to 15 each leg	60 s	106
B1. Knee-banded quadruped hip extension	2 to 4	10 to 15 each leg	0	109
B2. Knee-banded fire hydrant	2 to 4	10 to 15 each leg	0	117
B3. Knee-banded bodyweight glute bridge	2 to 4	10 to 15	60 s	102

Table 9.5 Glute Circuit 5

In sequence perform the A giant set of four exercises in sequence for the prescribed number of repetitions. Rest for approximately one minute between rounds. Then move to the B giant set and perform each exercise for the prescribed number of repetitions. Rest for approximately one minute between rounds.

Exercise	Sets	Repetitions	Rest	Page
A1. Dumbbell sumo squat	2 or 3	15 to 20	0	83
A2. Standing band hip hinge abduction	2 or 3	15 to 20	0	116
A3. Dumbbell hip thrust	2 or 3	15 to 20	0	106
A4. Bodyweight side-lying clamshell	2 or 3	15 to 20 each leg	60 s	112
B1. Single-leg glute bridge	2 or 3	15 to 20 each leg	0	103
B2. Ankle weight side-lying hip abduction	2 or 3	15 to 20 each leg	0	113
B3. Bodyweight reverse hyperextension	2 or 3	15 to 20	0	95
B4. Monster walk	2 or 3	15 to 20 each leg	60 s	111

CONCLUSION

Believe it or not, most of you will see tremendous progress in strength and physique without having to incorporate formal cardio into your regimen. Again, you'll want to let your diet and resistance training do most of the work. Most of you should use cardio as a secret weapon of sorts when you've maxed out all your other options.

The glute circuits may look unassuming on paper, but they'll give you a run for your money. The best part about them is that you can do them quickly, they're low impact, and they'll work your glutes—a three-in-one punch! I encourage you to tweak each circuit and substitute movements if they don't feel right to you or if you don't feel them working the appropriate muscles. For example, side-lying clamshells do nothing for my upper glutes, but seated hip abductions are my jam. Just be sure that the substitutions you make are from the same movement category.

ACTIONABLE ITEMS

- Ditch the cardio queen title and use the minimum effective dose approach. Keep cardio at a minimum to start and sprinkle in more on an as-needed basis. Let your nutrition and resistance training do most of the physique-sculpting work.
- Don't discount the effect that nonexercise activity thermogenesis can have on your daily energy expenditure.
- If you'd like to add some low-intensity, steady-state cardio, leisure walking may be a good choice for you, as it is for me.
- For a little bit of cardio with a twist, incorporate glute circuits into your routine. Perform 10- to 15-minute glute circuits two or three days a week.

PART

IV

Thrive

The final section of this book teaches you how to put all these moving pieces together. I've provided you with the tools you need to succeed, and here I'll show you how to put them to good use.

In chapter 10 I'll teach you how to write your own training program. You'll be able to create a workout regimen tailored to your individual needs, taking into consideration not only your training goal but also your time restrictions, equipment availability, exercise contraindications, and more.

Chapter 11 builds on chapter 10 and gives you the steps you need to put your plan into practice. I'll walk you through how to track your workouts, how to progress in the gym, and how to tweak the program to make it even better for you. I even provide some sample programs for you to follow, along with a dynamic warm-up.

The final chapter is all about monitoring your progress. How do you gauge how you're doing? When and how should you make changes to your regimen? I'll provide you with the information you need to assess your progress properly and accurately (rather than relying solely on scale weight) to determine whether you're moving in the right direction.

You have everything it takes to become your own coach. More than that, however, you have it in you to become the master of your own mindset, nutrition, and training journey. Let's forge ahead with the final steps.

CHAPTER 10

Create Your Program

Before I delve into the specifics of how to create your own training program, I want to clarify that there are an infinite number of ways to write sound programs that will yield results. I myself have tried dozens of ways of training. I've loved some, while others have left me dreading my sessions. Some programs made me feel as if I was doing a lot but ultimately did not get me any closer to my goal at the time. Conversely, I've scoffed at some programs on paper only to be humbled on the training floor and astonished by the changes that I've seen in my physique.

In this chapter, you'll learn to create your own training program. Even if you don't end up writing one for yourself, you should understand the hows and whys of your workouts. Doing so will give each exercise and set more meaning, and you'll know how to make adjustments and substitutions to your program when needed without having to rely on another resource.

Consider yourself a student of the gym.

TAKE INVENTORY

First things first: Take inventory of your logistics. After all, what good is a regimen that requires you to perform the leg press if you don't have access to the machine? Would it make sense to follow a program that requires you to be in the gym for six hours a week if you can afford only three?

Taking inventory is all about laying out the tools you have at your disposal before determining your plan of attack. What limitations do you face? What instruments do you have to work with? This important step will allow you to design a program that will not only maximize your time in the gym but also deliver the best results for you as an individual.

The good news is that no matter how busy you are, what equipment you have available, or what movements you can and cannot perform, you can create a well-designed program that will make you stronger, look better, and feel more confident.

TIME AVAILABILITY AND PREFERENCE

In an ideal world, you would have no time constraints with regard to your workouts. The gym would be a short commute away, and you'd have the freedom to train at the time of day that best suits you. You would be able to go through your workout at your leisure, not worrying about when you have to be back out the door and on to your next commitment.

The bad news is that most of us don't have unlimited time to spend in the gym. The good news is that with my training programs, you need only a few dedicated hours per week to see lasting results in your physique and strength.

Most of us are busy, and I respect that. Some of you are full-time students who also have full-time jobs. Maybe you're a mom whose children are involved in many activities, or perhaps your job is incredibly demanding and you feel as if you hardly have time to breathe. This is all fine.

My programs allow you to see results with even the busiest of schedules. All I'm asking of you is a small handful of hours per week to devote to building a stronger, more sculpted body.

My preference would be for you to lift weights three or four days per week, with maybe an extra hour or two for miscellaneous pastimes such as light walking. All told, then, you'd be looking at a maximum of six hours of per week, not including commute time to and from the gym.

But what about the minimum? If time is of the essence to you, then even an hour and a half per week—two 45-minute resistance-training sessions—can yield some spectacular changes, especially for a beginner trainee.

Can you afford that much time per week? If the answer is no, you should consider taking a hard look at how you spend your free time. Chances are you probably spend an hour and a half mindlessly scrolling social media—time that you could use to do some good old-fashioned hard work and sweat.

Science Plug

Many fitness buffs consider it common knowledge that a muscle group needs a minimum of 48 hours of rest after being trained (Kraemer et al. 2002). A survey of 127 competitive bodybuilders found that all 127—that is, 100 percent of them—used a body-part split, and two-thirds of them worked each muscle group just one day per week. Some argue, however, that performing fewer working sets per muscle per session may help decrease fatigue and, hypothetically, allow said muscle to be trained more frequently (Dankel et al. 2016). Why would this be beneficial? Dankel and colleagues (2016) predict that trained people may experience greater muscle growth by spreading their training volume over more sessions per week because they would be taking advantage of a hypothetical 24-hour refractory period and avoiding wasted sets (that is, extra sets that do not contribute to hypertrophy). Although this idea is new and no studies have yet been conducted to test it, it's something to consider when determining your training frequency, especially as you advance in your lifting career.

All told, most of you should reasonably expect to be in the gym on the training floor two to four days per week. Start here even if you could be in the gym more frequently. Many people make the mistake of diving in too quickly. They try to make the leap from years of living a sedentary lifestyle to becoming a workout fiend overnight. This approach, while admirable, is too much of a behavior change and is ultimately unsustainable. Drastic life overhauls rarely last. Begin with what you can stick to first and master that before tossing more variables into the mix.

EQUIPMENT AVAILABILITY

You don't need fancy, state-of-the-art equipment to complete my programs, but you do need some basic items. If you've been thinking about outfitting your own home gym, I strongly recommend doing so, particularly if you have the space and the means. I took the plunge a few years ago, and it's saved me a good deal of time (no commute!) and stress. Not having to wait to use a specific pair of dumbbells and not needing to wipe another person's sweat off the bench have alone made it worth it, but I also enjoy having the freedom to blast my own music and film exercise videos for me and for my clients with no hassle.

Decking out your home gym doesn't have to be an expensive project. All you need is a dedicated area of your home. You can start with a squat rack, barbell, and some plates. From there, add to your collection over time. You can cut costs by purchasing used equipment that's still in good condition. Otherwise, my preferred brands are Rogue, Sorinex, and EliteFTS.

If you belong to a commercial gym or are scoping out training facilities to join, you should look for a few particular items. Here's what I recommend:

Gym mats

Squat stand or power rack with chin-up bar

Barbell (ideally, the Texas Power Bar)

Weight plates and clips (bumpers ideal for deadlifting)

Squat Sponge or Hampton extra thick barbell pad (for hip thrusts)

Adjustable bench

Dumbbells (light, medium, and heavy pairs—maybe 5 pounds [2.3 kg], 15 pounds [6.8 kg], and 30 pounds [13.6 kg] to begin with)

Aerobic step with risers

Stability ball

Long resistance band

Miniband (such as the Hip Circle)

Gym chalk (to help with grip)

If you're looking for more fun toys to up your gym ante, consider investing in the following:

Hip thruster (hipthrustwithsohee.com)

45-degree hyperextension machine

Trap bar

Dumbbells and dumbbell rack

Kettlebells and kettlebell rack

Ankle weights

Fractional plates (such as the Iron Woody brand)

Dip belt (for weighted chin-ups)

TRX or Jungle Gym suspension training system

Landmine unit

Most commercial gyms have a plethora of machines including the cable pulley system, leg press, leg extension, leg curl, shoulder press, seated row, and chest press. These machines are great and can be programmed into a well-designed training regimen.

Of course, you can get creative with equipment. A bench can be used not only for bench press but also for chest-supported rows, hip thrusts, step-ups, Bulgarian split

Your Questions Answered

Q: Should I invest in any training accessories? I've seen women wearing belts and special shoes when lifting. Do I need those?

A: Beyond your standard workout outfits and shoes, you really don't need anything more. But the more strength focused among you might find that a few extra training accessories help your performance in the gym. First, you can invest in a quality weightlifting belt; I like the Iron Tank lever belt, although I've had good experiences with the Rogue Ohio buckle belt as well. For shoes, the Adidas women's powerlifting shoes and the Nike Romaleos are my choices for squatting and benching. I like flat-soled shoes such as Chuck Taylors for everything else. Finally, for knee support, you can grab some knee sleeves. But don't feel obligated to shell out your money for these accessories; these are luxuries, not necessities.

squats, and dumbbell pullovers. The lying leg curl and even the leg extension machine can be used for easy, convenient hip thrusting. A little thinking outside the box can uncover endless possibilities for exercise variety.

All is not lost if you, say, don't have a power rack or if your dumbbells only go up to a specific weight. You can substitute movements or make regular exercises far more difficult through techniques such as increasing time under tension, increasing range of motion, and decreasing the base of support.

INJURY HISTORY AND EXERCISE CONTRAINDICATIONS

An important yet often overlooked aspect of training-program design is nixing exercises that are contraindicated because of either injury or discomfort. Many coaches and fellow fitness aficionados may be quick to tell you that you absolutely must perform this exercise and that movement or you'll never see the results you're looking for. This advice couldn't be further from the truth.

One of my long-term clients, Lauren D., incurred a knee injury while performing lunges not long ago. She reached out to me and asked what she could do in the meantime while she nursed her knee back to health. I quickly figured out that squats, lunges, and other knee-dominant exercises were out. A set of bodyweight hip thrusts also induced some pain, which told me that for lower-body movements, she should stick to straight-leg hip-dominant exercises for at least a few weeks. I made sure she could work around the temporary exercise contraindications by programming cable pull-throughs, American deadlifts, back extensions, and plenty of lateral rotary work. She was able to maintain much of her lower-body muscle mass by hammering out those movements in the two months it took for her knee to feel better.

I had another client, Michelle K., who had undergone hip surgery a few years earlier. She was not allowed to deadlift more than 250 pounds (115 kg) and found that barbell hip thrusts always hurt her, no matter how much she tinkered with her form. No problem. She was able to drop her body-fat percentage and get absolutely shredded with me by nailing her diet in the kitchen and incorporating exercises such as lighter, higher-repetition deadlifts, barbell glute bridges, single-leg hip thrusts, back extensions, good mornings, squats, and lunges. Her exercise contraindications didn't hold her back from seeing the kind of progress she wanted.

What about shoulder issues? Many people report pain with full range of motion bench press and direct overhead movements such as military press and push press. If this is you, you can experiment with landmine press and floor press, and you may find that using a neutral grip (rather than a pronated grip) for your dumbbell upper-body pushing exercises feel much better.

The best course of action with an injury is to work around it and let your body heal rather than stubbornly try to push your way through the pain. This detour isn't the end of the world; it's an opportunity to get creative with your programming. In addition, this time offers you an opportunity to learn a specific exercise that you've been meaning to master or address a body part that you've been wanting to hone in on.

Even if you're perfectly healthy with no broken bones or nagging strains, some movements may not feel right for you and you may not enjoy them. We all have a handful of exercises that we despise for one reason or another. For me, I've always dreaded high-repetition band hip thrusts, frog pumps, and overhand grip pull-ups. This is more than fine! As I said before, you don't have to perform any specific exercises. You can do a multitude of equally effective exercises in the same movement category to maintain your progress in the gym.

As a general rule, if it hurts or feels off in any way, don't do it.

GOAL

Time and equipment availability aside, the details of a training program will be highly contingent on your ultimate fitness goal. Do you want to train for a powerlifting meet? Then your workouts should be centered on the squat, bench, and deadlift and structured so that you gain strength in the three movements over time.

Do you want to shed body fat and firm up all over? A general emphasis on the main compound movements in a variety of repetition ranges and a sprinkling of accessory work would make the most sense.

Do you want to grow the derriere? Then most of the exercises you perform should emphasize the glutes. You should perform plenty of movements for the lower glutes such as hip thrusts and lunges, as well as movements for the upper glutes such as lateral walks and seated hip abductions.

By identifying your ultimate desired destination, you'll be able to map out a strategic plan of attack.

PROGRAM DESIGN VARIABLES

Now that you've taken stock of what you have to work with, let's move on to specific program design variables. Here you'll start to identify the specifics of your workout regimen while staying within your unique parameters.

SPLIT

When people think of bodybuilding—or body sculpting in general—they most immediately look to body-part splits. This approach to training is indeed popular, but it's just one of several ways of going about your workouts.

With body-part splits, each workout is devoted to one or two specific body parts. Monday might be chest and back, Tuesday legs, Wednesday shoulders and arms, and so on. This method can come in handy with higher training frequencies, because you'll be giving your muscles ample opportunity to rest and recover between sessions. Typically, you work each muscle group just once a week with this approach.

You can also employ an upper–lower split, whereby you alternate between working your entire upper body in one session and your entire lower body in the next. This plan is ideal when lifting four days per week, because you can hit the upper body twice a week and the lower body twice a week.

Finally, a full-body split, or total-body split, entails working just about every muscle in your body each workout. This approach allows you to work each major muscle group three or more times per week.

Which method elicits the best hypertrophy results? A 2015 study by Schoenfeld and colleagues looked at the differences in muscular adaptation between training each muscle group once per week (body-part splits) versus three times per week with a total-body approach. All 19 subjects performed three sets of 8 to 12 repetitions per exercise, and training volume was equated between the two groups (Schoenfeld et al. 2015). After following an eight-week protocol, those using a total-body routine experienced greater increases in muscle mass in the biceps and a trend for greater increases in the triceps and quadriceps.

This result doesn't necessarily mean that a total-body routine is superior, and I'm not trying to recommend that you ditch your split routine immediately. One point to consider is that although weekly volume was equated in this study, in the real world, body-part splits tend to involve much higher per-workout volume. Therefore, including a higher-volume routine for the body-part split participants could easily have led to better gains.

Additionally, most of the subjects employed body-part splits before the study, so we can't rule out the novelty factor here. Simply switching up the training stimulus may have been sufficient to induce superior benefits. Had the subjects been on full-body routines before the study, the split-routine group may have come out on top.

My take on this issue is that just about every kind of training split has a place. Each approach has benefits and drawbacks. With a body-part split, you can obliterate one muscle group within a single training session, but you don't work it again until the following week—that's a lot of rest and not a lot of training frequency. With a full-body split, you end up hitting each muscle group with higher frequency, which can be better for maximizing muscle gains, but the workouts can be more fatiguing.

For women in particular, I like either a full-body or lower–upper split routine. Marci Nevin, a personal trainer in the Bay Area, also prefers the full-body split with her female clients, because she's noticed that women tend to respond better to high volume and recover faster from workouts. Additionally, full-body workouts in general often feel more challenging than, say, a whole day devoted to training just the biceps and triceps. This last point can be important in satisfying the need of many people for a training session to *feel* fatiguing to get results. In this way, you give your clients what they want while still giving them what they need.

FREQUENCY

As I mentioned before, my recommended training frequency is three or four days per week. Depending on what you have going on in your life and how the workouts make you feel, you may find that you're less run down and experience better strength gains in the gym with fewer sessions.

I do not recommend training five, six, or seven days a week for most people. From working with hundreds of female clients and experimenting with all kinds of training programs, I've noticed that most women do not perform as well and feel more tired when they do too many workouts.

Seeing the best results is not necessarily about training more, but rather about being smarter about how you use your time.

In general, the higher the training frequency is, the lower the volume each session should have. You also have more wiggle room to toss in accessory work because you have more opportunities to train. Conversely, with a two-day split, you should stick almost exclusively to the main compound movements and include more sets and total exercises per workout.

EXERCISE SELECTION AND ORDER

The movement that you want to prioritize should be programmed first in a workout. Seems pretty straightforward, right?

This principle can be in reference to either an exercise that works a specific body part the best for aesthetic purposes or a lift that you want to improve. For example, if I want to focus on building up my backside, I might program hip thrusts first on day 1, glute bridges first on day 2, and dumbbell back extensions first on day 3. Or I could program hip thrusts first for all three training days. Or I might toss in barbell hip thrusts first on day 1, high-repetition back squats for day 2, and band hip thrusts for day 3.

Be sure to include the following into each workout for improved glutes:

At least one bridge exercise

At least one squat exercise

At least one hinge exercise

At least one lateral rotary exercise

Or perhaps your goal is strength because you're a powerlifter. In that case, programing the following would make sense:

Squat exercise

Bench exercise

Hinge exercise

Any accessory movements you want to add

The possibilities are endless, but the themes remain largely unchanged across the board. In most instances, the primary compound movements should be programmed first, followed by accessory movements, and finally any single-joint exercises you'd like to toss in.

VOLUME

Volume is a measure of how much work has been performed. Training volume is quantified by the load multiplied by the number of repetitions multiplied by the number of sets performed in any given workout. Some fitness professionals like to define it in other ways, but the gist is the same.

A good deal of controversy surrounds the importance of volume in muscle growth and the amount of volume that is sufficient. Here's my take. More volume in the gym is better only up to a point. Genetics plays a big role in how much training volume is optimal for each person. I know women who can perform five heavy working sets of squats multiple days per week and make tremendous gains in strength this way. Others, however, would be crippled by the same approach.

Be careful not to become a volume addict. You can become hooked on the feeling of exhaustion, but don't confuse fatigue with progress.

You may find yourself rolling your eyes at my programs at first, claiming that you surely need more sets and exercise than what I have written out for you. You may think that you're too advanced for something like this or that you're a special snowflake. I hate to break it to you, but this is likely not the case.

Many people don't get stronger, and thereby don't make physique progress, because they fail to understand how volume integrates with effort. Some even combine several training programs, do everything under the sun, and then wonder why, a year later, they still look the same. It's not always about doing more.

Finally, not all volume is created equal. A set of heavy deadlifts is not the same thing as doing a set of seated hip abductions. The movements that work your muscles in the stretched position produce the most damage and therefore should be done with the least volume relative to anything else.

If you're smart about how you apply my training programs, chances are that the workouts will be more than enough for you.

As far as sets and repetitions, I typically prescribe 1 to 3 working sets of the main movements in the range of 1 to 10 repetitions. The heavier, low-repetition sets come first, medium-weight, medium-repetition (8 to 15) sets are next, and I wrap up my workouts with lighter, high-repetition (16 or more) sets.

Be honest with yourself. Are you the type to overdo things and grind out repetitions until a blood vessel is about to pop? Or do you tend to amble your way through a lift? If you are the former, you might want to stick with exactly what I've written or even cut back a set on each exercise. If you are the latter, an extra set of the accessory movements may be warranted.

You should do only as much volume as you can recover from. Of course, some degree of fatigue and soreness is normal, especially when you've just tried a new exercise or your training volume has spiked. But your workout should not negatively affect your quality of life in an appreciable manner; you should be able to go about your day-to-day activities with relative ease. Typically, recovery from a training bout should take approximately 48 hours. If you're run down for a prolonged time from all the sets you've been performing, you have to pull back. You should be feeling refreshed and ready to go for most of your workouts.

More is not better; better is better.

LOAD AND EFFORT

Load and effort are two related yet distinct concepts in the world of strength training.

Load is a specific, quantifiable value that can be defined as a percentage of your 1-repetition maximum (1RM) for an exercise. For example, if your current maximum deadlift for 1 repetition is 200 pounds (91 kg), then 75 percent of that load would be 150 pounds (68 kg). You can also define load by a repetition range, meaning that your bench press 10RM would be the weight you can lift for 10 repetitions with good form (and attempting the 11th repetition would end in either failure or form breakdown).

Effort is subjective and refers to the degree of exertion. How hard does a set feel to you, and how hard are you trying? That's what effort is. The two primary ways to measure effort are rating of perceived exertion (RPE) and repetitions in reserve (RIR), which recently has been gaining popularity. With RPE, you rate your level of exertion on a scale of 1 to 10, with 1 reflecting little to no exertion and 10 being the highest level of exertion possible. RIR, in contrast, is a measure of how many repetitions you have remaining at the conclusion of each set.

One of the criticisms of using load, or intensity of load, for specific sets and repetitions in strength training is that performance may vary from day to day; although you may have been incredibly strong in the gym last week, that may not be the case today (Steele 2014). Test administrator error can also lead to imprecise training prescriptions.

Regardless, load and effort are closely interlinked. Attempting to set a 1RM personal record, for example, will require your full effort. A 5RM set that was reasonably difficult last week may require more effort today if your sleep, stress, hydration, and nutrition have been subpar.

Save your high-effort sets for the major exercises: squat, deadlift, hip thrust, bench press, and chin-up variations. You can take these lifts to failure. Don't be afraid to pull back on effort, however, if you're having a particularly crummy day. For the medium- to high-repetition sets of the accessory lifts, you can use medium effort—stop one or two repetitions shy of failure. Finally, for isolation or lateral rotary movements, you can leave several repetitions in the tank.

Be smart about your training. You shouldn't be grinding out every single set in every workout. Be selective about how and when to exert high effort and when to focus more on feeling the muscle working.

TEMPO

The *tempo* of an exercise can be broken down into four components: the eccentric phase (lengthening muscle while contracting), the pause at the midpoint of the lift, the concentric phase (shortening muscle while contracting), and the pause at the end of the movement.

Tempo is denoted by four numbers in sequence. You'll typically see tempo written out as something like 3-0-1-0 or 3010. This notation means that for the squat, for example, you'll descend for 3 seconds, pause for 0 seconds at the bottom, take 1 second to ascend, and pause for 0 seconds at the top.

Rarely do I have my clients count their tempo as they perform their lifts, so don't worry about tempo too much. What I want you to focus on for most exercises is controlling the eccentric portion with a two- or three-second count rather than cranking out your repetitions as quickly as possible.

Of course, specific tempo is important at times, such as with the powerlifting-style bench press, which requires a pause at the bottom of the movement. For this exercise, you might have a 2220 tempo prescribed.

REST TIME

We love to feel fatigued in the gym. Many of us have been conditioned to believe that a workout is worthwhile only if we leave the training floor drenched in sweat and practically limping out the door. Many of us like to believe that the more tired we are and the more repetitions we do, the better results we'll see.

I've noticed over the years that women in particular tend to fear resting between exercises. During my time as a boot camp instructor and personal trainer, I've witnessed clients trying to do jumping jacks and even burpees between sets of heavy squats. Why? They'll be quick to say, "To burn more calories, of course!" But we should not be thinking of resistance training this way.

When it comes to creating a caloric deficit, your nutrition should be taking care of most of that. How, then, does lifting weights fit into the context of a body-sculpting fat-loss regimen?

"Everyone's worried about burning calories, but they overlook building muscle, strength, and confidence," says Dan Trink, cofounder of Fortitude Strength Club in New York City. "We've gotten to the point where, for women in particular, it seems to be all about chasing fatigue. People think that if they get tired, then they're improving their body composition—but this is not the case."

The purpose of training should be to retain or gain muscle mass (or strength). To do that, you need to use rest periods strategically throughout your workout.

Jogging in place or walking laps around the gym does not qualify as resting. This activity is counterproductive, because insufficient rest means that you won't be as strong during your working sets. You'll be pushing less weight for fewer repetitions than normal.

For the best strength and muscle gains, resting for three minutes between working sets is better than resting for one minute (Schoenfeld et al. 2015). Brad Schoenfeld believes that based on the current body of literature on rest periods, one minute of rest is insufficient to recuperate strength. Inadequate rest ultimately compromises volume load.

The length of the rest period also depends on what exercise you're working on as well as the number of sets and repetitions you're performing. In general, you should rest longer between sets for the compound movements in the range of 1 to 5 repetitions. For sets of 6 to 15 repetitions, 2 minutes is sufficient, and for sets with more repetitions, 30 to 90 seconds is good.

But don't get your panties in a twist about this. I used to be a stickler about my rest periods. I'd wear a digital watch for my workouts so that I could count my rest times down to the second. Being neurotic is not necessary and can take the enjoyment out of your sessions. Approximate rest times work just fine.

HYPERTROPHY STRATEGY

You may have been told that if you want to gain muscle, all you have to do is lift heavy weights. But the process of gaining muscle, also called *hypertrophy*, is a little more nuanced than that.

Schoenfeld (2010) proposed three mechanisms of hypertrophy that have since been widely accepted as the gold standard in the bodybuilding world. A training program must have three aspects: mechanical tension, metabolic stress, and muscle damage.

Mechanical tension, which refers to the load being lifted, is arguably the most important contributor to hypertrophy. Mechanical overload induces increases in muscle mass; unloading leads to muscle atrophy (Goldberg et al. 1974). In other words, setting PRs and lifting more weight over time will generate greater mechanical tension, which will help build more muscle.

Metabolic stress is the deep burning sensation or insane pump you get when performing an exercise for high repetitions or contracting a muscle like crazy. This sensation is brought on by a buildup of metabolites—lactic acid, hydrogen ions, inorganic phosphate, and so on—that accumulate in the body. In turn, this buildup leads to alterations in hormones, cell swelling, and anabolic transcription factors.

Muscle damage contributes to the delayed onset muscle soreness (DOMS) you may feel in the hours following an exercise bout. The damage is created when you perform an unfamiliar exercise (or one that you have not done in a long time), stretch a muscle under activation, or emphasize the eccentric (stretching while contracting) component of a movement. DOMS is believed to stimulate satellite cell activity, which then promotes muscle growth.

No single mechanism is sufficient for maximizing muscle hypertrophy. The most effective training programs include all three components through careful selection of exercise, set, and repetition.

Although we don't yet know the ideal combination of the three mechanisms, plenty of gains can be made by striving to get stronger in the major compound movements across a variety of repetition ranges and tossing in accessory work in the medium- and high-repetition ranges for the pump and burn.

PERIODIZATION

A few years ago, a fellow trainer wrote a post about how he planned his clients' periodization cycles 52 weeks in advance. He had a spreadsheet with every cell color coded, and he had included strength, hypertrophy, and endurance phases, as well as a special color for times when he knew his clients would be out of town. If anyone got sick or couldn't make a session for an unexpected reason, he said that he would sit down at his computer and modify the entire plan.

My eyes practically bulged out of my head. Mind you, these were general health and fat-loss clients, not professional athletes. Why make things so complicated?

Periodization, or the fluctuation of training stress, can be confusing and overwhelming, but I don't like to approach it that way, especially for everyday people like you and me who just want to look good and feel good.

Ben Bruno uses a top-secret proprietary system that has produced some jaw-dropping transformation for his clients within a matter of months. He uses a top-secret proprietary system that has produced some jaw-dropping transformations for his clients within a matter of months. Are you ready for it? He calls it life periodization. All jokes aside, that's essentially what I do for my clients as well.

When you're feeling good on any given day, push hard and try to set PRs. If you're feeling crummy—maybe you didn't get enough sleep last night or your nutrition has been shoddy—then pull back on your effort. If you have to go out of town and miss a few sessions, then you can count that as your deload, a dedicated period when you intentionally pull back on intensity in the gym to give yourself a physical and mental break. If you've been pushing the envelope in the gym for four to six weeks, you can program a deload period.

Contrary to what many people think, deloads are beneficial. Deloads typically last one week and involve a purposeful reduction in training load or volume. My general recommendation is to cut back on load by 40 to 50 percent and cut down on the total number of sets performed by up to 40 percent if you're feeling particularly fried.

You may fear that if you're not going all out with your workouts every single time and grinding yourself into the ground, then you'll stall your progress, or worse, lose precious muscle mass. But you need these periods for recovery, injury prevention, overall performance, and most important, training longevity.

I recommend using the first week of any new training program as a deload week. You can take advantage of this time to go lighter in weight and practice a new movement or an exercise that you haven't done in a while. Then, in the following weeks, you can increase your effort and chase strength.

Think of it this way: If you keep grinding week in and week out without hitting the brakes, eventually you'll be forced to deload because of an injury. A better approach is to take preventative measures and scale back regularly to keep your body fresh and chugging along over the long term.

Your Questions Answered

Q: Is there a best time of day to train to optimize results?

A: In general, physical performance appears to be worst in the early morning and best in the late afternoon. Research indicates, however, that training adaptations are specific to the time of day at which workouts are regularly performed (Hill et al. 1998; Chtourou and Souissi 2012). If you work out at, say, 6 a.m., after a few weeks your body will acclimate to perform well at that time. I have clients who do their training sessions at 4 a.m., whereas others wait until the evening crowd disperses to get their pump on. In short, the best time of day for you to work out is whatever will allow you to stick to a consistent schedule.

Q: I've been lifting weights for three months, but I don't look drastically different. What gives?

A: Gaining muscle is a painstakingly slow process, particularly for women. Most of us simply don't have the testosterone levels needed to support appreciable muscle growth. With that said, focusing on week to week or even month to month changes can be frustrating because it's hard to notice subtle short-term changes. Instead, I encourage you first to make sure that your nutrition is dialed in, because that aspect is the most important determinant of fat loss. Then do an honest audit of how your workouts have been going. Have you been showing up to the gym consistently? Have you been tracking your workouts and getting progressively stronger over time, or have you been merely going through the motions? If you've been dotting all your i's and crossing all your t's, then you're doing everything right. Learn to enjoy the process and celebrate any milestones, however small. Keep this up long enough, and the aesthetic changes will come in time.

ACTIONABLE ITEMS

- Before creating your training program, take inventory of your time availability and preference, equipment availability, injury history and exercise contraindications, and fitness goal.
- Identify your program design variables: desired training split, frequency, exercise selection and order (depending on your fitness goal), and volume.
- Be mindful of your load and effort. Plan to exert high effort for the major exercises and focus more on feeling the muscle working for the accessory and isolation lifts.
- Rest for up to three minutes for low-repetition (1 to 5) sets, two minutes for medium- repetition (6 to 15) sets, and one minute for high-repetition (16 or more) sets.
- Employ life periodization with your workouts: Push hard in the gym when you feel good and pull back when you feel crummy. Schedule program deloads every four to six weeks for recovery, injury prevention, overall performance, and training longevity.

CHAPTER 11

Sample Programs

Now that you've learned the fundamentals of writing a quality program, let's move forward and put the training wheels in motion. (Get it?)

In this chapter I'll discuss how to translate your program on paper into results in the weight room. I'll also include sample two-, three-, and four-day split programs that each last 12 weeks. Although you should choose the option that best suits your time availability and schedule, you'll see the best results by training three or four days a week.

Nevertheless, let's move forward with the details.

PUTTING IT INTO PRACTICE

Knowing how to put together a program is only half the equation. A plan written on paper means nothing unless it is properly executed.

In the following sections you'll learn the elements of carrying out your workouts not only to maximize results but also to do so in a way that leaves you feeling rejuvenated, rather than defeated, by your training sessions.

TRACKING WORKOUTS

For the first six years of my lifting career, I wasn't diligent about tracking my workouts from week to week. I would walk into the gym, try to remember what weights and repetitions I did the previous week, and then aim to match or beat that.

I didn't have a system. I couldn't flip back through my training journal—because, you know, I didn't have one—and say,

> *Ah ha! On February 14 I lifted precisely 185 pounds (84 kg) for three repetitions, and then on February 21 I pulled 195 pounds (88 kg) for three repetitions, but my notes indicate that this was a sloppy set and that I should stay at this same weight next week and work on getting better form.*

It wasn't until my seventh year of lifting that I realized my strength levels had more or less stalled after my first full year of resistance training. I rarely missed a session, and I pushed myself hard with each working set. But to my dismay, several years had gone by without noticing that my numbers had made no improvements.

In my naiveté, I thought I was smart enough to keep a mental log of my workouts and let that be sufficient. And I was wrong.

Learn from my mistake and track your workouts from the get-go. You can pick up a training journal from my online store, www.soheefit.com/store. I like the journal because it keeps all your sessions from any given month streamlined, and it's easy to see at a glance what you lifted in the previous weeks. Alternatively, you can spend a few dollars to buy a lined notebook and simply jot down the weight, sets, and repetitions performed for each exercise and any comments that might be useful in the future.

INDIVIDUALIZATION

Most of you will be able to follow the workouts provided in this chapter to the letter without a problem, but I encourage you to modify the program by up to 20 percent if needed to suit your individual needs.

You may find that although I prescribe, say, the barbell bench press, the gym that you frequent only has a bench press station that's rarely open at the time you usually go. You don't want to stand around and wait for 20 or 30 minutes when you could perform a similar variation, finish your workout, and be out the door in less than an hour. So grab a pair of dumbbells and perform the dumbbell bench press or even the dumbbell floor press. The muscles worked are virtually the same, and you'll be saving yourself precious time.

Or perhaps you find that side-lying clams just don't do it for you. It's an awkward exercise, and you don't feel your muscles much, if at all. If that's the case, pick another movement from the lateral rotary category in chapter 8 that you like and substitute it. The movements you perform should not only feel good and induce no pain but also have you feeling your muscles working in all the right places.

Pay close attention to the kinds of exercises your body likes. If your goal is gluteal hypertrophy, for example, then you need to be mindful of what squat pattern, hinge pattern, bridge pattern, and lateral rotary movements activate your glutes the most.

I've found that I don't really feel heavy barbell hip thrusts, and I do not enjoy high-repetition band hip thrusts at all. Pausing at the top of the bridging movement, however, fires my glutes like crazy, so I gravitate toward high-repetition barbell hip thrusts, low-repetition band hip thrusts with a pause at the top of each repetition, dumbbell hip thrusts, and dumbbell glute bridges, all for high repetitions and typically with a pause at the top of each repetition. These exercises absolutely torch my lower and upper glutes. And when I want to isolate my upper glutes, I don't feel side-lying clamshells much, but seated hip abductions have my cheeks a-burnin'.

Finally, I've found that some women feel better and their performance in the gym improves when they're doing fewer working sets as opposed to more. What I've noticed is that this typically tends to happen in those who go almost too hard in the gym with every set. If this means that you reduce the prescribed working set for a given exercise from three to two—or maybe even one—then so be it. By taking careful notes of how you feel after performing a given movement, you'll quickly pick up on trends in how different variables affect you, and you'll be able to make adjustments accordingly.

My client Jenny has been working with me for over two years now, and I've written over a dozen training programs for her. Through constant communication about how her workouts are going, how her strength is progressing in the gym, and how she's been feeling physically and mentally, I've learned that she feels her best and progresses the most with an ultra low-volume program. She is unique in this way. I regularly program just two or even one working set of maybe five or six exercises per training session for her and call it a day. Some might cry out that this volume is offensively low and that she couldn't possibly see any gains from this scant regimen, but she feels like a million bucks with this kind of regimen. She is continuing to see both strength and hypertrophy improvements over time. If this program works for her, why would we mess with the system?

You can achieve excellent physical results in many ways. Keep in mind that the programs written out here are just a starting point.

WEIGHT SELECTION

Every now and then, clients ask me to prescribe specific weights for them to use during their working sets. The problem is that everyone has a different strength level. Even as a beginner to the weight room, you may be able to bust out a set of squats with a weight that the person next to you has worked diligently for two years straight to hit. Conversely, the bench press may not be your forte, and you may be outpaced by a less-experienced, more petite person.

This circumstance is normal. Don't pick up a certain pair of dumbbells just because you saw someone else using them. This is about you, not anyone else.

Whenever you encounter a new exercise, or even when you're performing a familiar movement with a new number of prescribed repetitions, use your warm-up sets to gauge what your weights should be for your working sets. If possible, perform a few repetitions with just your body weight and adjust from there. Of course, you'll need to consider other variables such as your energy level for that day, which may influence your acute strength.

The weight you select depends highly on the prescribed number of repetitions as well as your prescribed effort (if applicable). In general, I recommend choosing a weight that allows you to perform the set so that one or two more repetitions would result in form breaking down. If you finish a set feeling as if you could have cranked out several more repetitions with ease, you should go up in weight for the following set. On the other hand, if you don't get anywhere near your prescribed repetitions before concluding the set early, your weight was too heavy.

You can perform *ascending sets,* in which the amount of weight you use for each successive set is heavier than the last; you can do *straight sets,* in which the weight for all working sets is the same; and lastly, you can perform *descending sets,* in which the weight you use decreases with each set you perform.

In most instances, I recommend sticking to either ascending sets or straight sets. Ultimately, what weight to use next is a judgment call on your part. How did the last set feel? Did it feel smooth, fast, and light? Do you think you could have easily performed several more repetitions? If the answer is yes, you should lift heavier weights; if the answer is no, use the same weight again.

Weight selection is a skill that will improve over time as long as you're paying attention.

PROGRESSIVE OVERLOAD

Getting to the gym and going through the motions with your workouts is not enough. This is how I went nowhere fast for six years,

In its simplest terms, progressive overload is doing more over time. Although progressive overload is traditionally thought of as adding more weight to the bar, it's much more than that. Improvement can occur in three primary ways.

Load

If you're a beginner to the weight room, a smart way to approach a new exercise is to use the lightest possible load. Usually, that means using just your body weight, the lightest pair of dumbbells available, or a barbell with no plates loaded. As a newbie trainee, much of your first few weeks in the gym will be about grooving the proper movement pattern and establishing neuromuscular control.

Over time, a given weight will become too easy for you, and you'll be able to progress by adding more resistance. You will be increasing mechanical tension, which, if you remember, is one of the three mechanisms of hypertrophy.

You are ready to go up in weight when you complete a set feeling as though you could have completed several more repetitions without batting an eyelash. With lower-body movements, you might tack on an extra 5 or 10 pounds (2.3 to 4.5 kg). For upper-body movements, you may find that your strength increases are incremental. This process is normal, because your upper-body muscles are a good deal smaller than those of your lower body.

One thing to keep in mind is that strength gains are not linear. If that were the case, then within one year your deadlift could skyrocket from, say, 135 pounds to 395 pounds (88 to 179 kg) just by going up by 5 pounds (2.3 kg) every week. Wow! Wouldn't that be nice?

Some weeks you will feel as if you're lifting on rocket fuel. All the weights that felt heavy before will be flying up as if they're nothing. This feeling is great, and I encourage you to take advantage of this time to push the boundaries and set PRs in the gym. Other times, however, you may find yourself in a rut; your numbers stay steady and don't increase at all for what seems like forever. You may have the occasional week when, for seemingly no reason, your repetitions don't feel as smooth as normal, and none of the exercises feels quite right for you.

Remember, this sensation doesn't necessarily mean you're getting weaker. A myriad of factors affect your strength levels from day to day, including but not limited to caloric intake, sleep and stress, training status, and more. And you can't forget the influence that genetics and underlying injuries have on your progress.

Don't focus on week-to-week or even month-to-month fluctuations in strength. Step back and look at the long-term trends. Are you stronger now than you were six months ago? How about one year? If the answer is yes, then you're doing something right.

Volume

You can progress by increasing your volume. Traditionally, when we talk about increasing training volume, we refer to doing more sets or repetitions, either within a set or within the scope of an entire training session.

Alternatively, you can incorporate more volume by increasing the frequency with which you train while leaving the per-session volume intact. For example, you might go from training three days per week to four days per week.

A concept related to volume is *time under tension*, which refers to the duration of a given working set. Increasing duration is a way to induce metabolic stress. To increase time under tension, you can perform more repetitions within a set or tack on more overall sets.

In addition, you can increase the *density* of a training session by decreasing the rest periods taken between sets. If you typically hip thrust 135 pounds (61 kg) for eight repetitions with three minutes of rest, but this week you can knock out 135 pounds for eight repetitions with two minutes of rest, you have successfully increased the training density and thus implemented progressive overload.

Range of Motion

If your squat goes up by 50 pounds (23 kg) in two months, but you've been cutting your squat depth shorter and shorter, can you really say you've gotten stronger? Conversely, if you were quarter squatting last month with 135 pounds (61 kg), but you can now do a below-parallel squat with the same 135 pounds, does that mean that you haven't progressed at all?

Concrete numbers are great when tracking workouts because they're straightforward, but they don't always tell the whole story. You need to be consistent with the form you use to execute a repetition and the range of motion you cover.

In general, always use a full range of motion, keeping in mind that a degree of individual variation is involved. Depending on injury history, mobility, and body structure, full range of motion can mean going to parallel for one person (because going any lower may induce hip pain), whereas the person next to her can squat all the way down with ease.

In this aspect, then, you can progress either by increasing range of motion with a given weight or by achieving the same range of motion and using more weight.

Exercise Progression

Finally, you can implement progressive overload by performing a more advanced version of an exercise. This method typically entails decreasing the base of support, increasing the demand on the body, or learning a more difficult skill.

Most people do not think of progressing an exercise as a form of progressive overload, but in a way, it is. You're placing muscles under extra stress and practicing a more difficult task.

You can regress or progress just about any exercise depending on your skill level. With the hip thrust, for example, you would want to master the bodyweight bilateral hip thrust first before progressing to the single-leg bodyweight hip thrust. When learning the push-up, you can start with the incline push-up, decrease the degree of incline as you gain strength until you work your way to the floor, and then move to the narrow-grip push-up.

DECIPHERING THE PROGRAMS

Now let's dive into the programs themselves. These workouts will get you progressively stronger, build confidence, and help you look better over time. Furthermore, they're efficient, meaning that you won't have to make exercise your part-time job. Each exercise has a special purpose, and nothing prescribed here is a junk movement. You'll get the most from your effort with these kinds of workouts, which incorporate all variations of the main compound movements across a wide range of repetition ranges.

Some of you who are new to the world of strength training may feel overwhelmed when glancing over the workouts. Although everything may seem to be written in a foreign language, the programs are pretty straightforward after you know how to read them.

EXERCISE ORDER

Perform the exercises in ABC order. You complete sets and repetitions of exercise A (taking the appropriate rest time between sets, of course) before moving to exercise B. A number following a letter in the exercise order column, such as A1 and A2, means that the exercise is a *superset*. You perform one set of A1, then one set of A2, and continue alternating between the two movements until you have completed all sets. If you have A1, A2, A3, then you have a *triset*, and you will cycle through the three exercises, performing one set at a time. A1, A2, A3, A4 is called a *giant set*, which involves four exercises in sequence. You get the idea.

REPETITIONS

Normally, you'll be prescribed a repetition range for an exercise, such as three sets of 8 to 12 repetitions. Select a weight or level of difficulty that you estimate will allow you to stay within the repetition range with good form. After you've completed all three working sets for 12 repetitions, make a note in your training journal to go up in weight or difficulty the following week. Aim to hit 8 repetitions per set and then work your way up again.

But don't be married to repetitions. If you can do 12 repetitions of the military press with the 45-pound (20 kg) barbell, but the next weight increment puts you at 50 pounds (23 kg) and you can perform only 6 repetitions (leaving you 2 repetitions shy of the allotted 8 to 12 range), that's alright. Forcing out extra repetitions with sloppy form and risking injury is not worth it. If you need to stop short, do so.

REST PERIODS

Unless otherwise noted, adhere to the following approximate rest recommendations:

For sets of 1 to 5 repetitions, rest three to five minutes.

For sets of 6 to 15 repetitions, rest two minutes.

For sets of 16 repetitions or more, rest one minute or less.

TRAINING TERMINOLOGY

Finally, I want to cover some terms and acronyms you may encounter. I've also included terms that you won't see mentioned here because I want to make this guide as comprehensive as possible.

I should note that in the programs that follow, I write out many of the acronyms in full to make the programs as clear as possible. But when transcribing exercise names into your training journal, you may eventually find it far easier to write out "SL DB HT" rather than "single-leg dumbbell hip thrust."

Here are some abbreviations and acronyms to familiarize yourself with:

Abd: abduction

Alt: alternating

APT: anterior pelvic tilt

BB: barbell

BSS: Bulgarian split squat

BW: bodyweight

CG: close-grip

CSR: chest-supported row

DB: dumbbell

DL: deadlift

KB: kettlebell

OH: overhead

HT: hip thrust

PPT: posterior pelvic tilt

PR: personal record

SB: stability ball

SL: single-leg

UG: underhand grip

WG: wide-grip

Singles means performing sets of one repetition, *doubles* refers to sets of two repetitions, and *triples* are sets of three repetitions. If you have three sets of three repetitions prescribed, you might say that you're doing three triples.

You'll see *AMRAP* mentioned a few times in my programs, which stands for "as many repetitions as possible." AMRAP is best used when you are performing bodyweight exercises or exercises with a specific weight prescription (for example, goblet squat with 45 pounds [20 kg]). You are to perform as many quality repetitions using a full range of motion as you can, and the goal is to do more repetitions each week.

Constant tension means keeping the muscles under constant tension through the duration of a set, typically by shortening the range of motion. You don't set the weight down or give yourself an opportunity to rest between repetitions. This approach is a great way to induce metabolic stress. I love to use the constant tension approach for the barbell hip thrust in particular, although it can be used with many other exercises as well.

With a *rest pause set*, perform as many quality repetitions as you can at a given load. Rest 5 to 15 seconds (some people like to denote a specific number of breaths to take, such as three to five). Perform more repetitions, rest, and continue in this manner until you have completed all the prescribed repetitions. You can squeeze in more volume at a heavier weight than you would otherwise be able to do.

Finally, a *drop set* is a technique in which you perform repetitions with a given weight, immediately reduce the weight, and continue to perform more repetitions until you reach failure. A variation of this is *running the rack*, in which you perform as many repetitions as you can with a pair of dumbbells, then pick up the next lighter pair of dumbbells and do as many repetitions as possible, and continue down the dumbbell rack. With barbells, this variation is called *plate stripping*, and it involves pulling plates off the bar between clusters of repetitions.

WARM-UP

Rather than walk into the gym and head straight to the nearest squat rack, take a few minutes to warm up. Some of you may be impatient and think that warming up is a waste of time, but this time allows you to increase your core temperature, increase your range of motion before heavy lifting, and activate your muscles. Perform both a general warm-up and a specific warm-up.

GENERAL WARM-UP

The general warm-up is a 5- to 10-minute routine performed before the workout begins. Besides preparing the body for the session ahead, the warm-up serves as a ritual to focus and visualize the upcoming lifts.

In the general warm-up, you want to perform dynamic stretches, in which you move as you stretch. Contrast this technique with static stretches, in which you stretch and hold a specific position for several seconds. Many people make the mistake of doing static stretches in preparation for their training session, but doing so may actually decrease muscular strength and power (Yamaguchi and Ishii 2005). Static stretches are better saved for either after the workout or in a separate session altogether (Behm and Chaouachi 2011).

You don't need to make the warm-up routine complicated. Perform a few key exercises and get on with your workout. Table 11.1 shows a sample warm-up that lights up the entire body and helps to work up a light sweat.

Of course, if you want to address a specific body part or movement pattern, be sure to incorporate that into your routine.

Some people will be fine doing less, but others will need to do more to feel sufficiently ready to train. Adjust according to your individual needs.

Table 11.1 Sample Warm-Up

Exercise	Sets	Repetitions	Page
Bodyweight glute bridge	1	20	195
Inchworm to hip lunge	1	5 per side	195
Push-up	1	5	196
Side-to-side leg swing	1	10 per side	196
Walking knee hug	1	10 per side	196
Dumbbell goblet squat	1	5	197

BODYWEIGHT GLUTE BRIDGE

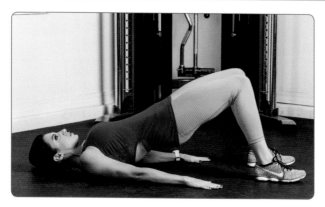

Figure 11.1 Bodyweight glute bridge.

Lie back into a supine position on the ground. Position the feet just outside shoulder width, flatten the lumbar spine, and place the heels on the ground with the knees at approximately a 90-degree angle. Extend the hips, pushing through the heels. Achieve full hip extension and squeeze the glutes at lockout. Lower the hips to the ground in a controlled manner.

INCHWORM TO HIP LUNGE

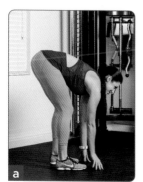 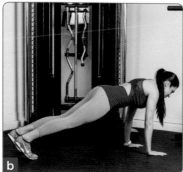 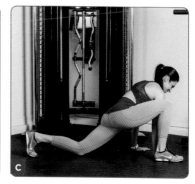

Figure 11.2 Inchworm to hip lunge: *(a)* starting position; *(b)* plank; *(c)* lunge.

From a standing position, reach down and touch the floor in front of the body with both hands. You should have a soft bend in the knees. Slowly walk the hands out until the body is in a plank position. Plant the right foot outside the right hand and sit the hips down. Then return to the plank position and repeat, planting the left foot outside the left hand. Slowly walk the hands back toward the body.

PUSH-UP

Start in a plank position with the arms extended and the body in a straight line. Place the hands just outside shoulder width on the floor. Keeping the head, neck, and spine in a neutral position, lower the chest to the floor and touch the chest to the ground. Tuck the upper arms at a 30- to 45-degree angle relative to the torso and keep the body in a straight line. Reverse the motion by pushing the body back up to the starting position.

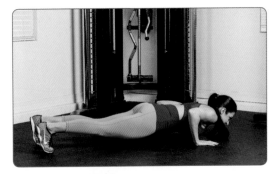

Figure 11.3 Push-up.

SIDE-TO-SIDE LEG SWING

Stand and face a power rack or something sturdy to hold onto for balance. With the right foot a few inches (cm) in front of the body, swing the right leg from side to side, using as much range of motion as comfortably possible. Repeat on the other side.

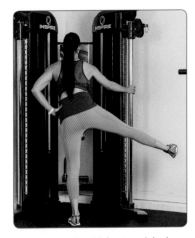

Figure 11.4 Side-to-side leg swing.

WALKING KNEE HUG

Stand and lift the left knee toward the chest and hug it into the body with both hands. Lower the left knee to the ground and take a step forward with the left leg. Repeat on the other side.

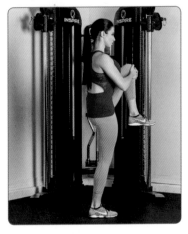

Figure 11.5 Walking knee hug.

DUMBBELL GOBLET SQUAT

Stand and hold one weight end of a dumbbell against your chest, resting the weight on your palms. Position your feet slightly wider than shoulder width and flare your feet out 30 to 45 degrees. Take in a deep breath and drop your hips straight down in a controlled manner while pushing your knees out and staying as upright as possible. Your elbows should stay between your knees at all times. Squat until your hip crease is in line with your knee joint or lower. Reverse the motion by pushing through your heels and squeeze the glutes to lockout.

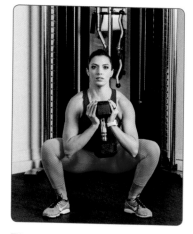

Figure 11.6 Dumbbell goblet squat.

SPECIFIC WARM-UP

The specific warm-up involves performing a few repetitions of a given exercise at a lighter weight before starting the working sets. Many women tend to do far too much for their warm-ups, thereby fatiguing themselves before even getting to the sets that count.

My approach is to do as little as needed to feel warm and ready to lift heavy weights. If you've been prescribed three sets of five back squats and you're planning to start your first working set at 135 pounds (61 kg), it may be sufficient to do five repetitions with the 45-pound (20 kg) barbell, rest two minutes, do three repetitions with 95 pounds (43 kg), rest two minutes, and then dive into your first actual set.

Treat every repetition of a warm-up set as if it were heavy. Don't simply go through the motions with complete disregard to form because you think it doesn't matter—it absolutely does! If anything, think of these repetitions as an opportunity to groove quality movement patterns and mentally prepare yourself for the heavy load ahead.

Of course, if you have an exercise with a greater number of repetitions prescribed, a warm-up set is not always warranted. For example, if you're doing two sets of 20 repetitions of lateral raises with a 5-pound (2.3 kg) dumbbell in each hand, do you really need to warm up beforehand? With what—1 pound (.45 kg) dumbbells? That approach seems a little excessive.

In general, the main compound movements should include one to three warm-up sets. With accessory movements, you'll likely be OK with just one warm-up set or none at all.

TRANSITION PROGRAM

The two-, three-, and four-days-per-week sample programs are written for people who have resistance-training experience with at least a moderate level of strength. How do you know if this is you? You should be able to perform most of the following with quality form:

20 bodyweight box squats to parallel or below

20 bodyweight hip thrusts

1 deadlift with 135 pounds (61 kg)

5 bodyweight push-ups from the floor

1 bodyweight chin-up

5 bodyweight bent-leg inverted rows

Everyone has a unique anthropometry, which may in turn affect your ability to perform some movements. Those of you with longer femurs, for example, may find that performing box squats to parallel is a particularly difficult task. And some women who have incredible lower-body strength have never been able to perform a single bodyweight chin-up because they have a muscular lower body and more mass in general. Don't sweat it if you're unable to execute one or two of these movements.

You have no reason to be embarrassed if you can't complete these exercises. Everybody has a unique starting point, and strength is a skill. The important aspect is to continue showing up for your workouts and focusing on quality form. In time, you'll be well on your way to squatting, deadlifting, and hip thrusting the big plates. If you can't complete the exercises, start with the transition program.

The transition program involves four days of training per week, and you should perform it for four weeks straight before moving on to the regular programs. I've designed this block so that you can perform all workouts from the comfort of your own home if you have a few pairs of light dumbbells, a couch off which to perform hip thrusts, and a chair for step-ups. You can get creative and find a platform in your home that will allow you to perform box squats to parallel, too.

The purpose of this phase is not only to build your strength and gain confidence in the gym but also to practice the main movement patterns until you can perform them well.

I recommend that you spread out your sessions. I would do a two-days-on, one-day-off, two-days-on, two-days-off schedule, like this:

Monday: day 1

Tuesday: day 2

Wednesday: off

Thursday: day 3

Friday: day 4

Saturday: off

Sunday: off

Alternatively, you could move your day 4 session to Saturday.

These workouts don't take long, which is entirely the point. From start to finish, each session should take you 30 minutes at most. By training four days a week, you'll have numerous opportunities to improve your motor control and gain confidence with the movement patterns. You should be itching to advance to the next phase of programs by the end of the four weeks.

I'm not trying to get you to leave the gym drenched in sweat, hobbling to the shower after every workout. You'll have a time and a place for that, and that time is not now. This phase is not about lifting egos; it's about priming your body to hoist some heavy weights.

Rather than simply go through the motions blindly, focus on trying to perfect the squat pattern, hinge pattern, and so on. If you're feeling particularly motivated, you can expedite your progress by busting out your camera and taking pictures of yourself performing exercises from the front and side angles. Eventually, strive for your hip hinge to look like the one shown in figure 11.7. Notice that the back is neutral or arched rather than rounded over and the shins are roughly vertical to the floor. The knees are bent softly, but this movement is hip dominant. One cue I like to give to help groove the hip hinge is to imagine that you're trying to tap a wall behind you with your butt.

Your squat should look like the one shown in figure 11.8. The squat involves a lot more knee flexion, but the back is still neutral or arched. The knees are pushed out, not forward, and the hip crease is in line with the knee joints. Going to parallel looks like this. You want to squat to this depth or below.

Don't forget that you get good at what you practice. Tables 11.2 through 11.5 outline the specifics of the transition program.

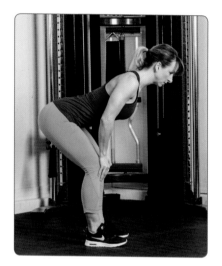

Figure 11.7 Proper hip hinge.

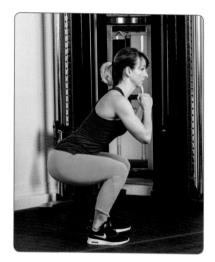

Figure 11.8 Proper squat.

Table 11.2 Transition Program Day 1

	Exercise	Sets	Repetitions	Notes	Page
A1.	Dumbbell single-leg Romanian deadlift	3	8 to 12 per side		97
A2.	Incline push-up	3	AMRAP	When you can perform 12 incline push-ups, decrease the degree at which your torso is elevated. Eventually, you should work your way to performing push-ups from the floor.	125
B1.	Bodyweight box squat	3	10 to 20	When you can perform 20 bodyweight box squats with ease, progress to the goblet box squat.	79
B2.	Chest-supported dumbbell row	3	10 to 20		131
C1.	Bodyweight glute bridge	2	20 to 30	When you can perform 30 bodyweight glute bridges with ease, progress to the dumbbell glute bridge.	195
C2.	Dumbbell military press	2	10 to 20		119

Table 11.3 Transition Program Day 2

	Exercise	Sets	Repetitions	Notes	Page
A1.	Bodyweight hip thrust	3	10 to 20	When you can perform 20 bodyweight hip thrusts with ease, progress to the dumbbell hip thrust.	106
A2.	Bent-leg inverted row	3	AMRAP		135
B1.	Bodyweight split squat	3	10 to 20 per side	When you can perform 20 bodyweight split squats per side with ease, progress to the dumbbell split squat.	84
B2.	Dumbbell bench press	3	10 to 15		121
C1.	Cable pull-through	2	10 to 15		92
C2.	Lat pulldown	2	10 to 15		128

Table 11.4 Transition Program Day 3

	Exercise	Sets	Repetitions	Notes	Page
A1.	Dumbbell Romanian deadlift	3	10 to 15	For this superset, use a pair of dumbbells light enough that you can perform both exercises with the same weight with ease.	96
A2.	Dumbbell floor press	3	10 to 15		122
B1.	Dumbbell goblet squat	3	10 to 15		197
B2.	Single-arm row	3	10 to 15 per side		133
C1.	Feet-elevated glute bridge	2	20	If you're feeling ambitious, wrap a miniband around your knees. This variation will light up your glutes.	104
C2.	Incline push-up	2	AMRAP	After you can perform 12 incline push-ups, decrease the degree at which your torso is elevated. Eventually, you should work your way to performing push-ups from the floor.	125

Table 11.5 Transition Program Day 4

	Exercise	Sets	Repetitions	Notes	Page
A1.	Bodyweight reverse lunge	3	10 to 20 per side	After you can perform 20 bodyweight reverse lunges per side with ease, progress to the dumbbell reverse lunge.	86
A2.	Seated row	3	10 to 20		130
B1.	Hip-banded hip thrust	3	20 to 30		106
B2.	Standing landmine press	3	10 to 20 per side		120
C1.	Bodyweight back extension	2	20		93
C2.	Cable Pallof press	2	10 per side		153

TWO-DAYS-PER-WEEK PROGRAM

This two-days-per-week program is perfect for those of you with incredibly busy schedules and limited opportunity to make the trip out to the gym or for those of you coming back from a training layoff.

I want to emphasize that training two days per week is not inferior to higher training frequencies provided you are smart about your programming. With these workouts (tables 11.6 to 11.11), you're still hitting the major compound movements in the low-, medium-, and high-repetition ranges. You can still make a tremendous amount of progress with this approach. You're in good hands!

Because you'll be strength training only twice a week, each session will have a little more volume than I would prescribe for a standard workout. To save time, however, I've supersetted the movements.

I recommend a Monday–Thursday, Tuesday–Friday, Wednesday–Saturday, or Thursday–Sunday schedule. This setup will give you three or four days of rest between the training sessions, so you'll feel refreshed and ready to go each time.

Table 11.6 Two Days a Week: Weeks 1 to 4, Day 1

	Exercise	Sets	Repetitions	Notes	Page
A1.	Barbell box squat	3	5 to 8	You may alternatively perform the dumbbell goblet box squat, in which case you should increase the repetition range to 10 to 15.	79
A2.	Seated row	3	5 to 8		130
B1.	Barbell Romanian deadlift	3	8 to 12		96
B2.	Dumbbell push press	3	8 to 12		119
C1.	Feet-elevated glute bridge	3	20 to 30	You may perform these knee-banded.	104
C2.	Bodyweight push-up	3	AMRAP	Regress to the incline push-up if your elbows are flaring out or if your butt is sagging when you do these from the floor.	125
D.	Cable Pallof press	3	10 per side		153
E.	Seated machine hip abduction	2	30	Use the seated hip abduction machine if you have access to one. Otherwise, the seated band hip abduction will work fine.	114

Table 11.7   Two Days a Week: Weeks 1 to 4, Day 2

	Exercise	Sets	Repetitions	Notes	Page
A1.	Barbell glute bridge	3	6 to 10	Use 25-pound plates on either side, if possible, in order to achieve more range of motion per rep. You may need a training partner to deadlift the barbell onto your lap.	101
A2.	Dumbbell floor press	3	6 to 10		122
B1.	Dumbbell reverse lunge	3	8 to 12 per side	Start with the weaker leg first, and then match the number of reps performed on the other side.	86
B2.	Single-arm row	3	8 to 12 per side		133
C1.	Bodyweight back extension	3	20		93
C2.	Half-kneeling landmine press	3	10 to 15 per side		120
D1.	Posterior pelvic tilt plank	2	10 to 20 second hold		150
D2.	Lateral walk	3	10 per side		110

Table 11.8   Two Days a Week: Weeks 5 to 8, Day 1

	Exercise	Sets	Repetitions	Notes	Page
A.	Barbell front squat	3	5		81
B1.	Barbell hip thrust	3	6 to 10		105
B2.	Band-assisted chin-up	3	5 to 8	If you are unable to perform the band-assisted chin-up, instead perform the inverted row or underhand-grip lat pulldown.	127
C1.	Good morning	3	6 to 10		94
C2.	Close-grip bench press	3	10 to 15	If equipment limitation is an issue, you may alternatively perform the flat dumbbell bench press.	124
D1.	Bodyweight quadruped hip extension	2	20 per side	You may perform these knee-banded, with the knee of the non-working leg anchoring the band to the floor.	109
D2.	Bodyweight side-lying clamshell	2	10 per side		112

Table 11.9 Two Days a Week: Weeks 5 to 8, Day 2

	Exercise	Sets	Repetitions	Notes	Page
A.	Deadlift	3	5		99
B1.	Dumbbell step-up	3	6 to 10 per side		88
B2.	Barbell military press	3	5 to 8		118
C1.	Dumbbell back extension	3	10 to 15		93
C2.	Barbell bent-over row	3	10 to 15		134
D1.	Bodyweight single-leg hip thrust	2	AMRAP		107
D2.	Fire hydrant	2	20 per side	You may perform these knee-banded.	117

Table 11.10 Two Days a Week: Weeks 9 to 12, Day 1

	Exercise	Sets	Repetitions	Notes	Page
A.	Barbell back squat	3	3		82
B1.	Barbell glute bridge	3	8 to 12	Use 25-pound plates on either side, if possible, in order to achieve more range of motion per rep. You may need a training partner to deadlift the barbell onto your lap.	101
B2.	Seated row	3	6 to 10		130
C1.	Stiff-legged deadlift	3	6 to 10		98
C2.	Barbell bench press	3	6 to 10		121
D.	Knee-banded barbell hip thrust (constant tension)	3	20	Rest 90 to 120 seconds between sets.	106

Table 11.11 Two Days a Week: Weeks 9 to 12, Day 2

	Exercise	Sets	Repetitions	Notes	Page
A.	Deadlift	3	3		99
B1.	Hip-banded hip thrust	3	8	Add a pause at the top of each repetition.	106
B2.	Bodyweight push-up	3	AMRAP	Perform the incline push-up if your elbows are flaring out or if your butt is sagging when you drop to the floor.	125
C1.	Dumbbell Bulgarian split squat	3	8 to 12 per side		90
C2.	Bodyweight pull-up	3	AMRAP		127
D1.	Frog pump	3	20		108
D2.	Standing cable hip abduction	3	10 per side	You have the option of performing this exercise with a band or ankle weight.	115

THREE-DAYS-PER-WEEK PROGRAM

Training three days per week (tables 11.12 to 11.20) is my sweet spot, and I suspect that it may be right up your alley as well. I love this training frequency for multiple reasons. Devoting just a few hours to the gym per week offers me more time and energy to focus on other aspects of my life. Because I always get at least two full days of rest between lifts, I not only feel energized for each session but also am that much more motivated to push it hard.

If I ever have to miss a session, I can simply shift my training schedule back by a day without having it disrupt my life.

Table 11.12 Three Days a Week: Weeks 1 to 4, Day 1

	Exercise	Sets	Repetitions	Notes	Page
A.	Barbell front squat	3	5		81
B.	Barbell bench press	3	5		121
C.	American deadlift	2	5 to 8		97
D.	Tall-kneeling single-arm cable pull-in	3	10 to 15 per side	If equipment limitation is an issue, you may alternatively perform this exercise with a long resistance band.	129
E.	Dumbbell single-leg hip thrust	2	10 to 15 per side		107
F.	Cable upright row	2	15 to 20		137
G.	Seated machine hip abduction	2	20	If equipment limitation is an issue, you may alternatively perform this exercise knee-banded.	114

Table 11.13 Three Days a Week: Weeks 1 to 4, Day 2

	Exercise	Sets	Repetitions	Notes	Page
A.	Deadlift	3	5		99
B.	Barbell military press	3	5 to 8		118
C.	Dumbbell glute bridge	2	30		102
D.	Seated row	3	8 to 12		130
E.	High step-up	2	6 to 10 per side	Start with just bodyweight, and when that is easy, progress to holding a 5 or 10 pound (2.3 or 4.5 kg) dumbbell in each hand.	89
F.	Incline dumbbell fly	2	15 to 20		141
G.	Monster walk	3	10 per side		111

Table 11.14   Three Days a Week: Weeks 1 to 4, Day 3

	Exercise	Sets	Repetitions	Notes	Page
A.	Barbell hip thrust	3	8		105
B.	Bodyweight chin-up	3	AMRAP	If you are unable to perform the bodyweight chin-up, instead perform the band-assisted chin-up, inverted row, or underhand-grip lat pulldown.	126
C.	Knee-banded dumbbell goblet squat	3	10 to 15		80
D.	Barbell incline press	3	8 to 12		123
E.	Bodyweight back extension	3	30	If you are unable to perform 30 consecutive reps, instead perform 3 sets of 20 reps.	93
F.	Dumbbell pullover	2	10 to 15		144
G.	Ankle weight side-lying hip abduction	3	10 per side		113

Table 11.15   Three Days a Week: Weeks 5 to 8, Day 1

	Exercise	Sets	Repetitions	Notes	Page
A.	Barbell glute bridge	3	8	Use 25-pound plates on either side, if possible, in order to achieve more range of motion per rep. You may need a training partner to deadlift the barbell onto your lap.	101
B.	Landmine row	3	5 to 8 per side		132
C.	Barbell box squat	2	5 to 8		79
D.	Close-grip bench press	3	5 to 8		124
E.	Dumbbell single-leg Romanian deadlift	2	8 to 12 per side		97
F.	Face pull	2	15 to 20	These may be performed from a seated or standing position.	145
G.	Standing band hip hinge abduction	2	15		116

Table 11.16   Three Days a Week: Weeks 5 to 8, Day 2

	Exercise	Sets	Repetitions	Notes	Page
A.	Deadlift	3	5		99
B.	Dumbbell push press	3	8 to 12		119
C.	Dumbbell hip thrust	2	20	Pause for a count of three at the top of each repetition. On the last repetition, squeeze the glutes at lockout and hold for as long as possible.	106
D.	Bent-leg inverted row	3	AMRAP	If you can perform 10 reps with ease, progress to the feet-elevated inverted row.	135
E.	Leg extension	2	15 to 20		154
F.	Dumbbell lateral raise	2	20		136
G.	Lateral walk	2	20 per side		110

Table 11.17   Three Days a Week: Weeks 5 to 8, Day 3

	Exercise	Sets	Repetitions	Notes	Page
A.	Barbell hip thrust	3	5		105
B.	Band-assisted pull-up	3	6 to 10	If you are unable to perform the band-assisted pull-up, instead perform the inverted row or overhand-grip lat pulldown.	128
C.	Barbell split squat	3	6 to 10 per side		125
D.	Narrow-width push-up	3	AMRAP		84
E.	Cable pull-through	2	10 to 15		92
F.	Straight-arm pulldown	2	10 to 15		143
G.	Bodyweight side-lying clamshell	3	10 per side		112

Table 11.18   Three Days a Week: Weeks 9 to 12, Day 1

	Exercise	Sets	Repetitions	Notes	Page
A.	Barbell back squat	3	3		82
B.	Barbell push press	3	5 to 8		119
C.	Stiff-legged deadlift	2	6 to 10		98
D.	Bodyweight chin-up	3	AMRAP		126
E.	Bodyweight single-leg hip thrust	2	AMRAP	If you are unable to perform the bodyweight chin-up, instead perform the band-assisted chin-up, inverted row, or underhand-grip lat pulldown.	107
F.	Dumbbell curl	3	10 to 15 per side		148
G.	Seated band hip abduction	2	20, 20, 20	Perform 20 repetitions leaning forward, 20 repetitions upright, and 20 repetitions leaning back.	114

Table 11.19   Three Days a Week: Weeks 9 to 12, Day 2

	Exercise	Sets	Repetitions	Notes	Page
A.	Deadlift	3	1		99
B.	Barbell bench press	3	3 to 5		121
C.	Dumbbell deficit reverse lunge	2	8 to 12 per side		87
D.	Chest-supported dumbbell row	2	8 to 12		131
E.	Knee-banded feet-elevated glute bridge	3	20		104
F.	Dumbbell skull crusher	3	10 to 15		147
G.	Knee-banded fire hydrant	3	10 per side	Anchor the miniband to the ground with the knee of the non-working leg.	117

Table 11.20   Three Days a Week: Weeks 9 to 12, Day 3

	Exercise	Sets	Repetitions	Notes	Page
A.	Barbell hip thrust	3	3	Add a pause at the top of each repetition.	105
B.	Barbell bent-over row	3	5 to 8		134
C.	Dumbbell walking lunge	2	8 to 12 per side		85
D.	Dumbbell floor press	3	8 to 12		122
E.	Bodyweight back extension	3	20 to 30		93
F.	Hollow body hold	3	10 to 20 second hold		151
G.	Standing ankle weight hip abduction	2	15 per side	You have the option of performing this exercise with a band or cable.	115

FOUR-DAYS-PER-WEEK PROGRAM

The four-day split (tables 11.21 to 11.32) entails two lower-body sessions and two upper-body sessions per week. I like this approach because although you have greater training frequency, you're still giving your muscles ample time to rest between workouts. You could create an equally effective full-body four-day split, but I wanted to give you some variety.

In the interest of saving time, many of the upper-body exercises have been supersetted. I've paired noncompeting movement patterns (for example, an upper-body push exercise and an upper-body pull exercise) so that your strength is not negatively affected. For the most part, lower-body exercises are to be done one at a time. Because lower-body movements tend to be more taxing, I want you to take full rest periods between working sets.

With this program, you're really working your glutes only two days a week. This frequency is fine, but some of you may want more. You have the option of adding one of the glute circuits from chapter 9 to the end of your upper-body session if you'd like, or you can simply toss in one or two higher-repetition sets of your favorite glute exercises. I'd probably choose the seated machine hip abduction and the bodyweight back extension, but the choice is yours.

I recommend a training schedule that allows three days of rest between upper-body sessions and four days of rest between lower-body sessions. Something like this schedule would work well:

Monday: lower body

Tuesday: upper body

Wednesday: off

Thursday: lower body

Friday: off

Saturday: upper body

Sunday: off

If this doesn't work for you, then a two-days-on, one-day-off (Monday–Tuesday–Thursday–Friday, for example) schedule is fine as well.

Table 11.21   Four Days a Week: Weeks 1 to 4, Day 1, Lower Body

	Exercise	Sets	Repetitions	Notes	Page
A.	Barbell box squat	3	5		79
B.	Barbell hip thrust	3	6 to 10		105
C.	Stiff-legged deadlift	2	8 to 12	Focus on feeling a stretch in the hamstrings rather than pushing to increase load.	98
D.	Dumbbell reverse lunge	2	8 to 12 per side		86
E.	Bodyweight back extension	3	20		93
F.	Seated band hip abduction	2	30		114

Table 11.22 Four Days a Week: Weeks 1 to 4, Day 2, Upper Body

	Exercise	Sets	Repetitions	Notes	Page
A.	V-handle lat pulldown	3	5		129
B1.	Barbell incline press	3	6 to 10		123
B2.	Chest-supported dumbbell row	3	6 to 10		131
C1.	Dumbbell push press	2	8 to 12		119
C2.	Seated row	2	8 to 12		130
D1.	Bodyweight push-up	2	AMRAP	If you are unable to perform the bodyweight push-up, instead perform the incline pushup.	125
D2.	Face pull	2	15 to 20	These may be performed from a seated or standing position.	145

Table 11.23 Four Days a Week: Weeks 1 to 4, Day 3, Lower Body

	Exercise	Sets	Repetitions	Notes	Page
A.	Barbell hip thrust	3	8		105
B.	Kettlebell goblet squat	3	8 to 12	If equipment limitation is an issue, you may alternatively perform the dumbbell goblet squat.	80
C.	Kettlebell deadlift	2	10 to 15	If equipment limitation is an issue, you may alternatively perform the dumbbell Romanian deadlift.	100
D.	Single-leg glute bridge	2	AMRAP		103
E.	Knee-banded reverse hyperextension	2	20		95
F.	Bodyweight side-lying hip abduction	2	AMRAP		113

Table 11.24 Four Days a Week: Weeks 1 to 4, Day 4, Upper Body

	Exercise	Sets	Repetitions	Notes	Page
A.	Barbell bench press	3	5		121
B1.	Seated row	3	5 to 8		130
B2.	Dumbbell military press	3	8 to 12		119
C1.	Straight-arm pulldown	2	8 to 12		143
C2.	Incline dumbbell fly	2	10 to 15		141
D1.	Bent-leg inverted row	2	AMRAP	If you can perform 10 reps with ease, progress to the feet-elevated inverted row.	135
D2.	Dumbbell lateral raise	2	20		136

Table 11.25 Four Days a Week: Weeks 5 to 8, Day 1, Lower Body

	Exercise	Sets	Repetitions	Notes	Page
A.	Barbell hip thrust	3	5	As you go heavier in load, be sure to keep the chin tucked and ribs down and achieve full hip extension with each rep.	105
B.	Barbell front squat	3	6 to 10		81
C.	American deadlift	2	8 to 12		97
D.	Goblet Bulgarian split squat	2	8 to 12 per side		90
E.	Dumbbell frog pump	2	20		108
F1.	Dumbbell back extension	3	10 to 15		93
F2.	Lateral walk	3	20 per side		110

Table 11.26 Four Days a Week: Weeks 5 to 8, Day 2, Upper Body

	Exercise	Sets	Repetitions	Notes	Page
A.	Barbell military press	3	5		118
B1.	Band-assisted chin-up	3	6 to 10	If you are unable to perform the band-assisted chin-up, instead perform the inverted row or over-hand-grip lat pulldown.	127
B2.	Dumbbell floor press	3	8 to 12 per side		122
C1.	Landmine row	2	8 to 12 per side		132
C2.	Cable upright row	2	10 to 15		137
D1.	Dumbbell pullover	2	10 to 15		144
D2.	Prone rear delt raise	2	15 to 20		139

Table 11.27 Four Days a Week: Weeks 5 to 8, Day 3, Lower Body

	Exercise	Sets	Repetitions	Notes	Page
A.	Sumo deadlift	3	5		100
B.	Barbell glute bridge	3	10	Use 25-pound plates on either side, if possible, in order to achieve more range of motion per rep. You may need a training partner to deadlift the barbell onto your lap.	101
C.	Dumbbell step-up	2	8 to 12 per side		88
D.	Lying leg curl	2	10 to 15		156
E1.	Bodyweight quadruped hip extension	3	15 to 20 per side		109
E2.	Knee-banded fire hydrant	3	15 to 20 per side		117
F.	Hollow body hold	3	10 to 20 second hold		151

Table 11.28 Four Days a Week: Weeks 5 to 8, Day 4, Upper Body

	Exercise	Sets	Repetitions	Notes	Page
A.	Barbell bent-over row	3	8		134
B1.	Close-grip bench press	3	8 to 12	If equipment limitation is an issue, you may alternatively perform the flat dumbbell bench press.	124
B2.	Tall-kneeling single-arm cable pull-in	3	10 to 15 per side	If equipment limitation is an issue, you may alternatively perform this exercise with a long resistance band.	129
C1.	Barbell push press	2	8 to 12		119
C2.	Single-arm row	2	15 to 20 per side		133
D1.	Hammer curl	3	10 to 15		149
D2.	Dumbbell skull crusher	3	10 to 15		147

Table 11.29 Four Days a Week: Weeks 9 to 12, Day 1, Lower Body

	Exercise	Sets	Repetitions	Notes	Page
A.	Barbell back squat	3	5		82
B.	Dumbbell single-leg Romanian deadlift	3	8 to 12 per side		97
C.	Hip- and knee-banded hip thrust	2	20	Add a pause at the top of each repetition.	106
D.	Dumbbell walking lunge	2	8 to 12 per side		85
E.	Cable pull-through	2	10 to 15		92
F.	Standing ankle weight hip abduction	3	10 per side		115

Table 11.30 Four Days a Week: Weeks 9 to 12, Day 2, Upper Body

	Exercise	Sets	Repetitions	Notes	Page
A.	Bodyweight chin-up	3	AMRAP	If you are unable to perform the bodyweight chin-up, instead perform the band-assisted chin-up, inverted row, or underhand-grip lat pulldown.	126
B.	Barbell incline press	3	6 to 10		123
C1.	Seated row	3	6 to 10		130
C2.	Prone rear delt raise	3	10 to 15		139
D1.	Face pull	2	10 to 15		145
D2.	Narrow-width push-up	2	AMRAP	If you are unable to perform the narrow-width push-up, instead perform the standard push-up or incline push-up.	125
E1.	Dumbbell curl	2	8 to 12		148
E2.	Rope triceps extension	2	8 to 12		146

Table 11.31 Four Days a Week: Weeks 9 to 12, Day 3, Lower Body

	Exercise	Sets	Repetitions	Notes	Page
A.	Deadlift	3	3		99
B.	Barbell hip thrust	3	5		105
C.	Barbell deficit reverse lunge	2	8 to 12 per side		87
D.	Dumbbell back extension	3	8 to 12		93
E.	Dumbbell glute bridge	2	30 to 50	On the last repetition, squeeze the glutes at lockout and hold for as long as possible.	102
F.	Standing band hip hinge abduction	3	20		116

Table 11.32 Four Days a Week: Weeks 9 to 12, Day 4, Upper Body

	Exercise	Sets	Repetitions	Notes	Page
A.	Barbell bench press	3	5		121
B.	Chest-supported dumbbell row	3	6 to 10		131
C1.	Barbell military press	3	6 to 10		118
C2.	Single-arm row	3	8 to 12 per side		133
D1.	Incline dumbbell fly	2	10 to 15		141
D2.	Feet-elevated inverted row	2	AMRAP	If you are unable to perform the feet-elevated inverted row, instead perform the bent-leg inverted row.	135
E.	Cable Pallof press	3	10 per side		153

ACTIONABLE ITEMS

- Start with the transition program if you need to. Otherwise, choose from the two-, three-, or four-day-a-week programs.
- Vary the prescribed programs by up to 20 percent to suit your individual needs. Tweak exercises according to the equipment available or what your body likes, and reduce the training volume if you feel run down.
- When choosing a weight for your working set, stick to a load that will allow you to go heavy while still maintaining quality form. If in doubt, err on the side of too light for your first set and adjust from there.
- Track your workouts from day 1. Be sure to note not only the exercises you perform but also the weight and repetitions for each set as well as comments about how the movements feel.
- Ensure that you make progress over time by improving your load, volume, range of motion, or exercise progression.

CHAPTER 12

Monitor Your Progress

Now you have all the tools you need to master your mindset, nutrition, and training craft. No doubt you're eager to get the wheels in motion. That's great, but now I want to equip you with the knowledge that you need to become your own coach.

How do you assess your progress? What do you look for, and how do you tell whether you're on the right track? When do you make changes rather than keep the program the same? If you've stalled, how do you know whether you should hit your workouts harder, pull back on your calories, or simply get a better night of rest?

This chapter will cover all of that and more.

GAUGE PROGRESS

If your goal is to shed body fat or gain muscle, you must have check-ins with yourself regularly. Numbers, data points, and pictures all play a role in giving you a comprehensive assessment of your progress. We can progress at three levels: aesthetic, performance, and quality of life.

AESTHETIC ASSESSMENT

Accurately assessing changes in your physique is perhaps the most difficult task, so we'll address that first. Many women make the mistake of judging their progress solely by changes to scale weight, which can be incredibly misleading and frustrating.

I'm going to teach you the facets that you should consider. I use this exact system with myself as well as with my clients, and it will equip you to be your own coach.

Body Weight

Many women tell me that the number blinking back at them on the scale in the morning determines how their day is going to go. If the number is low, they're beaming with joy and feel like Superwoman all day long; if the number is higher than they'd like, they feel defeated.

I've noticed many individuals have taken a liking to demonizing the scale. Fitness enthusiasts left and right proudly proclaim that they've chucked their scales in the trash. Colleagues and followers alike offer cheers of approval. "Don't let the scale control you!" they say. "Throw it out. It's evil!"

Ironically, the act of having to restrict your access to scale weight is proof that the implement controls you. It doesn't have to be this way, and it shouldn't.

The number on the scale controls you only as much as you allow it to. If you ask me, throwing out the device does not solve the problem; it avoids it. It's a form of procrastination. What happens the next time you're at the doctor's office for your annual checkup and the nurse practitioner instructs you to step on the scale? Do you throw a fit, refuse to cooperate, and act offended? Do you have a meltdown right there on the floor?

Scale weight is an incredibly valuable tool. The key is to have a mature relationship with the scale so that you can take the emotion out of the equation and interpret it within proper context rather than have a knee-jerk reaction.

Understand that a lower scale weight could be indicative of fat loss, but it could also be a reflection of dehydration. If you clock in higher one morning, the number might mean you've gained body fat, but it also might mean you've gained muscle, that you consumed more sodium than usual the night before, that you didn't get enough sleep, or any number of other explanations.

Before doing backflips in celebration or sobbing into your pillow, take a beat to do an honest audit of how the past month, week, and day has gone for you.

I don't agree that self-weighing every day is necessarily unhealthy. Of course, it can be if you're doing so out of fear or neurosis. But at the end of the day, it's simply one data point.

Whether you choose to step on the scale once a day, once a week, or hardly ever is up to you as long as the scale weight is not controlling you. If you're actively chasing a physique goal, however, I recommend self-weighing once every two weeks at the absolute minimum.

Body Circumference Measurements

Next up is body circumference measurements. Few people I know take the time to use a flexible tape measure and write down the circumference of their waist, hips, thighs, chest, and arms once every two weeks. But you don't want to skip this crucial step.

At the very least, take your waist measurement. I like to place the tape measure around the narrowest point on my torso; for me, that's right around my belly button (figure 12.1). For the hips, thighs, and chest, go around the largest area; for your arms, measure at the midpoint between your shoulder and your elbow.

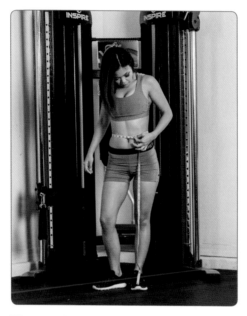

Figure 12.1 Waist measurement.

Don't worry too much about where the correct placement is for each point. What's important is being consistent from one check-in to the next.

Fit of Your Clothes

How have your clothes been fitting? Are your favorite pair of jeans sitting loose at the waist, or do you have trouble pulling them up by the hips?

Men and women alike frequently report feeling as if they're swimming in their clothes when they're shedding body fat. Conversely, they may sheepishly confess that over the winter, they've taken to donning hoodies and sweatpants because their usual tops and bottoms are a little snug. These tactile indicators are not to be ignored.

When you know, you know.

Progress Pictures and the Reflection in the Mirror

Measurements are certainly helpful, but they don't tell the whole story. You lose body fat in more than just the handful of places on your body at which you take measurements, and you have to consider human error.

Often my clients feel discouraged because despite dropping an inch (a few centimeters) off the waist and several pounds (a kilogram) off the scale, they'll look in the mirror and not see any visual progress. At this point I like to bring up the paper towel analogy (toilet paper works, too, but we'll stick with paper towels). You start with a full roll, and every day you pull off one or two sheets. You know you're reducing the number of paper towels left on the roll, but you can't see it yet. Eventually, though, you notice that pulling off one sheet at a time has added up, and you're now left with a much thinner roll than when you started.

Progress pictures and changes in the mirror can be useful here. Taking progress pictures regularly—once every two weeks if your goal is fat loss or muscle gain—is key to tracking long-term progress over time. Often my clients lament their lack of progress and complain that their physique changes have been happening too slowly. They might comment that they feel as if they've been spinning their wheels until I show them a side-by-side comparison of their starting photos versus current photos. I'm usually met with a startled, "Oh."

I recommend taking pictures every two weeks under the same conditions: first thing in the morning on an empty stomach after going to the bathroom, in a predetermined location under consistent lighting, in the same outfit (I recommend shorts and a sports bra or a bikini). In a relaxed position, get full body shots from the front, side, and back (figure 12.2). Keep these photos in a folder on your phone or your laptop so that you can track your visual progress throughout your fitness journey.

Even if you don't notice visible progress from week to week, don't immediately take that as a sign that you've stalled. Being completely subjective when it comes to physique transformations is impossible, so you have to take into account that some body dysmorphia may be happening, whereby you have a distorted image of your physical self (Pope et al. 1997). Typically, this effect is exacerbated the deeper into the dieting process you go (Rosen and Ramirez 1998). Be aware of this influence and know that it can compromise your ability to see yourself accurately.

Additionally, you'll notice that some days you feel like a lean bean and other days you could swear that you're backtracking, even though you're doing everything right.

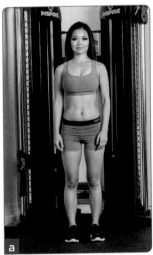 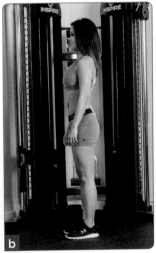 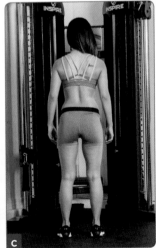

Figure 12.2 Progress photos: (*a*) front; (*b*) side; (*c*) back.

These day-to-day and even week-to-week fluctuations can result from changes in sodium intake, digestion, food sensitivities, stress, and much more. Try to stay levelheaded and don't freak out over short-term variations. Long-term trends are far more important.

Don't scrutinize your physique too much. Take the progress pictures and, rather than study every last detail on your body, tuck them away and move on with your day.

As a wise person once said, "Day by day, nothing changes, but when you look back, everything is different."

Comments From Others

The feedback you receive from friends, family, and coworkers is one of the most over-looked measurements of progress. Yes, this evidence is subjective, and yes, I think you should take all comments about your physique with a grain of salt, but if enough people are telling that you look leaner, then you can be pretty sure you're losing body fat.

Why do I love this form of assessment? Because someone who doesn't see you every minute of the day is going to more readily notice changes in your body than you are.

One caveat, however: Please do not let the insensitive remark of *one* person bring you down. Although unsolicited feedback on your body is often complimentary and welcomed, sometimes people can be straight up rude and hurtful. When people are making nasty comments, they are revealing their own insecurities. It has nothing to do with you.

Your body is yours alone. How you choose to look is nobody's business but your own. Nobody else's preference should matter, and how they think you should look shouldn't influence you. What matters most at the end of the day is that you're healthy, first and foremost, and that you are happy with your body.

A healthy emotional detachment is warranted here. Feedback is just that—feedback. Nevertheless, if others are noticing your progress, you can be sure that things are moving in the right direction.

PERFORMANCE ASSESSMENT

Now let's move on to performance assessment. Even if you don't consider yourself an athlete, keeping tabs on how you're doing physically can tell you a lot about how you're using your time in the gym.

Strength in the Gym

Whatever your fitness goal is, you need to chase strength in the gym. A mistaken idea floating around is that you should lift heavy if you want to gain muscle and get bulky, and you should stick to high repetitions and light weights to shed body fat.

Everyone should be striving to get stronger. Even if you want to get lean. Even if you want to look smaller and more petite. What builds the muscle, keeps it, after all.

Look through your training log and see whether you've gained strength in the main compound movements (squat, bench, deadlift, hip thrust, and chin-up) from month to month. Keep in mind that week-to-week fluctuations in strength are normal.

Figure 12.3 shows how my strength levels changed over the course of several months during my first powerlifting prep for the conventional deadlift. Notice that even though it looked as though I got weaker some weeks, over the long term I ended up with a net strength gain.

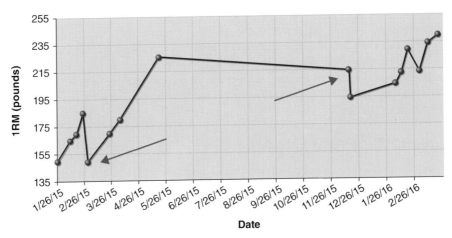

Figure 12.3 Conventional deadlift progression over time.

Your Questions Answered

Q: When you say we should be striving to get stronger, do I have to improve strength in every exercise every month? And if I'm not, does that mean that I'm not on the right track?

A: Not at all. Strength fluctuates considerably, and having to scale back the load by 20 pounds (9 kg) on the barbell one day doesn't necessarily mean that you've lost true physical strength. A number of variables influence strength, including but not limited to diet, hydration, electrolyte balance, sleep, and stress. Even when you've seemingly done everything right to prepare for a stellar session, you may find that you simply don't have it in you that day. Rather than look at one workout in isolation, focus on week-to-week and month-to-month progressions. Some weeks you may stall, some weeks you may seemingly move backward, and some weeks you may feel invincible in the gym. Take all this in stride and remember that you're on a journey. Strength gains are not linear!

When looking at your training progress, pay attention to the specific load used for each repetition range as well as any comments. Recall the various ways to implement progressive overload. For example, did you complete a set of squats with the same weight and repetitions as last month but with better depth? Did you keep your chin tucked and achieve full hip extension with your barbell hip thrust this time? Congratulations; you've made progress!

Bloodwork

Of course, we can't forget your actual physical markers of health. Blood tests are useful for evaluating how well your organs are working as well as assessing your risk factors for diseases. They can also provide a comprehensive metabolic analysis and give a snapshot view of your overall health.

Have your blood pressure and heart rate decreased? Have your cholesterol and insulin sensitivity improved? If so, you're on the right track.

These markers are more important than how lean and muscular you look. Although physical health tends to improve as body fat goes down, at some point getting too lean can be detrimental.

Overall Energy and Fatigue

You should notice that daily physical tasks that were once difficult are now easy to do. You've become a one-trip wonder when hauling groceries into your home from your trunk, whereas before you didn't have the strength to carry so much at once. When a kind gentleman asks you whether you need help lifting your carry-on bag to the overhead compartment on the airplane, you shake your head no because you've totally got this, baby!

Additionally, you want to be refreshed, not beat up, for most of your workouts. You should have enough energy to function outside the gym without an issue. For the most part, your fitness regimen should have you feeling more energetic and less fatigued than before.

I should mention that some mild fatigue and hunger are a normal and expected part of the fat-loss process. The longer you diet and the steeper your caloric deficit is, the more run down you're going to feel. You should try to keep this feeling to a minimum.

QUALITY OF LIFE ASSESSMENT

Finally, examine your quality of life. Remember how I told you about how I completely neglected this aspect at the beginning of my fitness journey? It cost me dearly. I alienated myself from my friends, I snapped at my family members, and my social life eventually dwindled down to nothing.

What's the point of being lean if you've become an unhappy wench in the process? Is having abs worth it if no one wants to hang around with you anymore?

For a long time, my answer to those questions was yes, I'm embarrassed to say. I had allowed myself to be so consumed with obtaining a particular physique that I let everything else in my life fall by the wayside. I was completely missing the point! I may have gotten lean, but I was not healthy.

That experience taught me a valuable lesson. Although I can't redo those years, I can use that experience to improve and help others. Don't let this happen to you.

Some of the fittest people you know may also be the most miserable. This link is not an accident. They've adopted extreme behaviors just to maintain their muscular, ripped bodies, but they've paid a price in terms of general life satisfaction. They likely don't get out much, and they spend most of their time in the gym. They'd rather stay home and doggedly stick to their homemade meals that perfectly fit their nutrition programs. That way they have complete control over their food.

Although they look physically fit and healthy on the outside, they may be unbalanced in their everyday lives. Lean does not always equal happy.

Here are some questions to ask yourself:

Have I been sleeping more soundly?

Am I happier and more confident than before?

Am I flexible enough to make adjustments to my training and nutrition program when needed without stressing out?

Can I attend a social function and enjoy myself?

Fitness should add to, not take away from, your quality of life.

MAKE ADJUSTMENTS TO YOUR PROGRAM

By now, you should have multiple data points as well as a solid pulse on how you've been doing in terms of aesthetics, general health, performance, and quality of life. From the plethora of information now at your fingertips, how do you know whether to make adjustments, and if so, what kind?

IF IT AIN'T BROKE, DON'T FIX IT

One error I see many people make with their programs is adjusting variables when they have no need to do so. If you've started out on the right foot with your training and nutrition—lifting weights a few days per week while getting stronger over time and finding a nutrition strategy that works for you—and you've been making good progress, then nothing needs to be modified. Keep doing what you're doing and don't mindlessly slash calories for no real reason.

I like to use the example of my client Andrea H. to illustrate my point. She came to me with the goal of shedding body fat, so I took over the reins of her diet. For a record 16 straight weeks, she was able to drop body weight and body circumference measurements and look visibly leaner check-in after check-in without a single adjustment to her nutrition program. She continued to lean out on the plan I had laid out for her. Why would I fix what wasn't broken?

Eventually, we reached a point where her progress stalled. At that point I finally dropped her calorie intake by a smidge, and she was able to continue making headway in her fat-loss endeavors.

I encourage you to take this approach. Don't change your program unless doing so is absolutely warranted. If you've got solid momentum going toward where you ultimately want to be, leave everything as is and keep trucking along.

The one exception to this rule is with training programs, which I recommend switching up every four to six weeks. With that approach, you'll prevent boredom in the gym and perform different exercises in different repetition ranges that will hit your muscles from different angles and continue to elicit a training effect.

In general, however, tweak the program only if something isn't working. For fat loss, this might mean that you haven't dropped measurements in several weeks. For strength gain, might mean that your squat 1RM hasn't budged in three months. Or it might mean that even though you're looking the best you ever have, you've become nasty, negative, and shallow. These signs all indicate that the system is no longer working and that you need to make a correction.

MAKE ONE CHANGE AT A TIME

Think of the scientific method. If you want to understand a process better, you manipulate only one variable while holding everything else constant. By controlling for all other variables, you can hone in on the influence of one factor on that outcome. If you have two or more variables that change at the same time, you won't know what exactly did the trick.

When it comes to making changes to your fitness program, the approach is the same. Make one change at a time and no more.

Table 12.1 Cheat Sheet for Interpreting Progress

Scale weight	Measurements	Strength	Potential meaning
No change	No change	No change	No change
No change	No change or increase	Increase	Increased lean body mass
No change	No change or decrease	Decrease	Calories too low
Decrease	No change or decrease	No change or increase	Lower body fat with retention of or increased lean body mass
Decrease	No change or decrease	Decrease	Lower body fat with decreased lean body mass
Increase	No change or decrease	Increase	Increased lean body mass
Increase	Increase	Increase	Increased body fat or increased lean body mass

In table 12.1 I provide a cheat sheet of sorts for interpreting and making sense of your progress. I encourage you to spend a few minutes looking over each line. This table is not comprehensive, but it's a solid starting point. You'll want to refer to this later when you do your own check-in to determine what steps, if any, to take next when tweaking your program.

In most cases, you'll be better off manipulating only one variable rather than two or three. Why? Because, as with the scientific method, if you change more than one thing at a time, you won't be able to put two and two together and deduce that one thing directly influenced another.

Rather than blindly choose one variable to change, however, be strategic about how you go about doing this. Figure 12.4 illustrates my hierarchy of physique changes.

Mastering the lower-level tiers will make a far bigger difference in your physique than focusing on the upper-level tiers. You should look first to your nutrition, then inspect the details of your training, and then examine your sleep and stress levels before considering sprinkling in extra cardio or conditioning.

Think of it this way: No matter how incredible your workouts might be and regardless of how soundly you've been sleeping this month, those aspects will make little difference in your fat-loss efforts if you've been eating like a glutton. You can't out-train a poor nutrition program—believe me, I've tried!

Here are some potential ways to adjust your program.

■ If your goal is fat loss and you haven't shed any body fat in several weeks, take a look at your nutrition. Go back and review chapter 5. Consider whether you have strayed from any living-lean guidelines. If you have, pick one behavior that you can tackle. If you're unsure about your nutrition intake, keep a food log for three days; write down everything you eat. Are you mindlessly consuming snacks throughout the day that you can cut? Have you started eating straight out of the bag instead of pouring the chips into a bowl? Are you not feeling satiated after meals? If you're not, can you ensure that you're consuming sufficient protein and fat per meal? Can you eat fewer but larger meals to help you feel fuller?

■ If you're trying to gain strength and muscle, first make sure you're eating enough food. Running on fumes will unnecessarily affect your performance in the gym, which

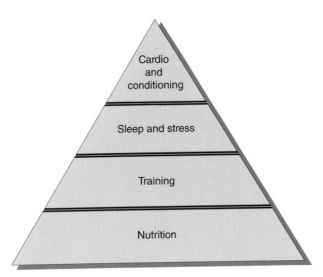

Figure 12.4 Hierarchy of physique changes.

will then compromise your ability to grow muscle. Next, check the specifics of your program design. Go back to chapter 10. Do your workouts incorporate all elements of a sound regimen, or is something missing? Are you approaching each session with high effort? Do you feel recovered by the next workout? Are you successfully implementing progressive overload? Are you resting enough and keeping your stress levels low to support strength and muscle growth? If not, what can you do in your life to change that?

■ If you're fit but your life outside the gym is in shambles, take a good, hard look at what might have gone wrong. Have you turned down so many social events in a row that you've stopped receiving invitations to hang out? Have you taken your dieting too far? Are your workouts no longer fun? Has that in turn made you crabby and moody?

■ If you're seemingly doing everything right—eating the right amount of calories and sufficient protein, training smart (and hard!) in the gym, and getting stronger over time—and everything that *should* be happening in the way of aesthetic progress simply is not coming to fruition, consider your sleep and stress levels. I have worked with numerous clients who, after making an active effort to cut down on the stress in their life and get a few nights of quality sleep, have experienced a whoosh effect, whereby they seemingly drop several pounds (a kilogram or more) of body fat overnight. Juma I. of Iraki Nutrition reports dropping 5 pounds (2.3 kg) off the scale in one day after months of stalled progress after finally taking an afternoon off work to decompress and getting a full night of rest. Yes, the effects of chronically elevated cortisol can be a huge obstacle—one that many people overlook. Rather than always try to push harder and grind the pedal to the metal, consider taking some time to chill out and rejuvenate.

■ If all your ducks are in a row but you're having trouble consistently executing the plan, the new behavior changes you're attempting to implement are not practical for you. Remember to start with small steps. You should always be striving for that intersection between behaviors (figure 12.5) that are practical (what you can and are willing to do consistently) and behaviors that are ideal (what will get you results). If you're doing what is practical but not ideal, you won't see lasting results because your daily behaviors won't get you closer to your goal; if you're doing what is ideal but not practical, the plan will look perfect on paper but adherence will be an in issue.

Don't get greedy and try to do too much at once. Doing so will only exacerbate the problem and further prolong your timeline.

Tackle one adjustment to your program for a minimum of two weeks before assessing your progress again. You can continue to follow the steps outlined in this chapter over and over, tweaking every two weeks or so if you need to.

BEWARE OF MINDSET TRAPS

No matter how prepared you think you are for your fitness journey, mindset traps will come knocking on your door. Most of you will find that despite your motivation in the beginning, you reach a point at which even the simplest task feels impossibly hard.

You may have come upon what is known as the hot–cold empathy gap, the inability to appreciate or gauge how difficult or uncomfortable a future situation will be (Loewenstein 2005). When you're well fed, well rested, and otherwise in a comfortable state, you mistakenly assume that you will always feel this way, even when the going gets tough. For that reason, many people set lofty fat-loss New Year's resolutions and fail. We commit to doing things in the future that we regret when the moment comes.

Even if you think you have what it takes to ward off adverse side effects that come with focusing on your physique, you're probably not immune. Beware of these potential mindset traps:

■ **Body dysmorphia:** You look in the mirror and even though you've made visible progress, even though body circumference measurements are dropping left and right, you don't think you look good. No amount of fat loss or muscle gain is quite enough, and you always want a little more. This perception is especially common among competitive bodybuilders or those trying to reach ultralow levels of body fat.

■ **Neurosis:** You're a nervous Nellie about going out to eat, about missing workouts, about scale weight. You might become anxious about social events and may even avoid them altogether. You might check your abs over and over in the mirror, checking to see whether your obliques are indeed popping out. Or is your mind just playing tricks on you? Or maybe it's the lighting. You may or may not find yourself slapping away your significant other's hand when he reaches for a bite of your food.

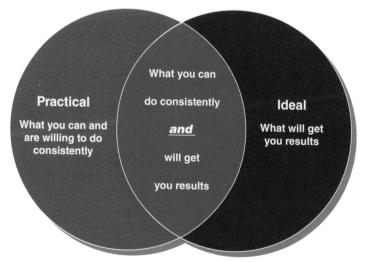

Figure 12.5 Progression sweet spot, the intersection of practical and ideal.

■ **Negativity:** You focus on all the things that are *not* going the way you want—your belly fat is still there, your arms still have too much jiggle, your booty isn't poppin' just yet. When a coworker comments that you're looking leaner, looking really healthy, you brush her off and insist that you still look horrible, even though you're down 10 pounds (4.5 kg) on the scale and your hips are down 2 inches (5 cm).

■ **Impatience:** If you lose half a pound (a quarter kilogram) of body fat in a week, you're frustrated that it wasn't twice as much. If you lose an inch (2.5 cm) off your waist in a month, you're upset that it wasn't three inches (7.5 cm). Despite the fact that it took you five years to reach your all-time highest body-fat percentage, you expect results overnight!

Being objective is incredibly, excruciatingly difficult when it comes to playing the fat-loss game. Even harder is keeping a solid head on your shoulders and taking the emotion out of the equation. Therefore, when monitoring progress, you should never look at one metric in isolation. I urge you to do a gut check every few weeks.

Body circumference measurements, scale weight, progress pictures, the fit of your clothes, comments from others—take all these factors into consideration, as well as any confounding variables such as dietary adherence, sleep and stress, digestion, sodium, menstrual cycle, and so on.

A hefty dose of emotional maturity is required to shed body fat or gain muscle without losing your cool and to maintain those results over the long haul. Don't obsess over the number on the scale. Keep tabs on all variables ensure that things don't spiral out of control.

FOCUS ON THE BIG ROCKS

At the beginning of my lifting career, I took great delight in combing through fitness online forums and quietly reading through all the threads on training and nutrition. I was eager to learn, but I allowed myself to become distracted by the plethora of information available. I quickly lost sight of the big picture.

Every three days, I'd change my nutrition program based on some new article I'd read online. First, it was all about carbs, and then it was all about fats (protein, of course, was always ultrahigh—the higher, the better!). I remember in particular someone asking in a forum whether almonds were a fat-loss food. A popular member of the board responded, "Yes, absolutely, you should have a whole handful a day!" The very next morning, I was popping into my mouth as many almonds I could fit into my hand, giddy that I had been lucky enough to stumble across the ultimate fat-loss formula in an obscure online discussion board.

Obviously, that plan didn't work. The serving size was ridiculous for someone my size, and I didn't stop to consider that one snack in isolation would not make or break me. I was majoring in the minors.

Don't let this be you. You may consider it a point of pride to be detail oriented, and it may well be, but not if you're becoming myopic and losing sight of the big picture in your fitness journey. Debating over whether broccoli or kale is healthier is focusing on small pebbles. Arguing about whether five or six repetitions of the back squat will yield superior strength gains is not worth your time. Which is better—30 grams of protein per meal or 40? These issues are the wrong ones to torment yourself with.

Focus on the big rocks. In his book *The Power of Habit: Why We Do What We Do in Life and Business*, Charles Duhigg (2012) calls these behaviors *keystone habits*. When mastered, these behaviors will have the biggest positive effect on your health and fitness.

Eat whole foods most of the time, train regularly while striving to get stronger from month to month, manage your sleep and stress levels, and enjoy your everyday life. That's the gist of it.

EAT, LIFT, AND THRIVE

I've lost count of how many programs I've forced myself to stick to, even when the thought of getting to the gym to do my workout filled me with dread and my prescribed meals made me gag. I'd feel anxious about my upcoming lifting session all day long, and I'd let out a huge sigh of relief when I'd finally finish my last set of exercises. I'd grit my teeth and choke down my dry chicken breast, half cup of broccoli, and six almonds while fantasizing about all the cake, ice cream, and cookies I couldn't wait to eat when my diet ended.

In other words, rather than look forward to my workouts and get excited about my meals, I was in a constant state of distress because of my fitness regimen. Within a matter of months—sometimes, mere days—I would jump ship. Then, discouraged by my slipup, I would deem the rest of the week a failure and stuff myself with junk food, vowing to do it right the next time. That was no way to live.

At the end of the day, what's the point of all this if you're not having fun? Your food should taste good, and your training should be fun. Most important, you should enjoy what you're doing and build momentum toward success.

I've said this before and I'll say it again: There are a million and one ways to put together an effective program. No one formula will fit everyone.

After you've mastered the big rocks, you can move on to the pebbles—the little details. How you choose to customize and tweak the finer points of your regimen is up to you. If you're staying injury free, seeing results, and having a good time, you're doing it right.

Like the way you eat.

Like the way you train.

The size of the wins doesn't matter as much as the fact that you're building momentum in the right direction. Find a way to keep the positive momentum going, no matter how small the wins.

Those who see the best results over the long term are the ones who rarely bounce from one extreme to another. Instead, they're really good at practicing moderate health behaviors while gently nudging themselves in the direction they want to go. They don't slash calories; they don't overdo it on the cardio; they don't try to go from zero to hero overnight. They show up day after day and month after month and do the work.

If you ever find yourself lost and overwhelmed at any point in this process, go back to working on mastering previous lessons from this book. There's no rush.

The joy in this whole journey is that you always have something to learn, always have another way to grow and improve your current self. Never can you declare that you've made it to the top and can no longer better yourself.

May you eat well, lift heavy and hard, and thrive in all aspects of your life for the rest of your days.

ACTIONABLE ITEMS

■ When assessing aesthetics, establish a healthy, nonemotional relationship with the scale. Regardless of how often you choose to weigh yourself, scale weight can be a useful data point when assessing progress. In addition, take body circumference measurements and pay attention to the fit of your clothes, the reflection in the mirror, and the comments you receive from others about your physique.

■ When assessing performance, examine your strength gains in the gym, bloodwork, overall energy and fatigue, and quality of life.

■ Don't make changes to your program until progress stalls or something goes awry. When you do make adjustments, modify one aspect of your program for a minimum of two weeks before assessing your progress again.

■ Beware of the mindset traps: body dysmorphia, neurosis, negativity, and impatience.

■ Focus on the big rocks of your fitness and don't fuss over the small pebbles.

REFERENCES

Alhassan, S., S. Kim, A. Bersamin, A.C. King, and C.D. Gardner. 2008. Dietary adherence and weight loss success among overweight women: Results from the A to Z weight loss study. *International Journal of Obesity*, 32(6): 985-991.

American College of Sports Medicine. 1990. Position stand on the recommended quantity and quality of exercise for developing and maintaining cardiorespiratory muscular fitness in healthy adults. *Medicine and Science in Sports and Exercise*, 22: 265-274.

Amos, C. 2013. The new pin-up: Why gentlemen prefer buff. http://nypost.com/2013/12/05/the-new-pin-up-why-gentlemen-prefer-buff.

Andrew, B.R. 1903. Habit. *American Journal of Psychology*, 13(2): 121-149.

Aragon, A.A., and B.J. Schoenfeld. 2013. Nutrient timing revisited: Is there a post-exercise anabolic window? *Journal of the International Society of Sports Nutrition*, 10(1): 5.

Aronson, E., and Mills, J. 1959. The effect of severity of initiation on liking for a group. *The Journal of Abnormal and Social Psychology*, 59(2): 177.

Bandura, A. 1982. Self-efficacy mechanism in human agency. *American Psychologist*, 37(2): 122.

Baumeister, R.F., E. Bratslavsky, M. Muraven, and D.M. Tice. 1998. Ego depletion: Is the active self a limited resource? *Journal of Personality and Social Psychology*, 74(5): 1252.

Behm, D.G., and A. Chaouachi. 2011. A review of the acute effects of static and dynamic stretching on performance. *European Journal of Applied Physiology*, 111(11): 2633-2651.

Bellisle, F., and A.M. Dalix. 2001. Cognitive restraint can be offset by distraction, leading to increased meal intake in women. *American Journal of Clinical Nutrition*, 74(2): 197-200.

Benedict, C., M. Hallschmid, A. Lassen, C. Mahnke, B. Schultes, H.B. Schiöth, J. Born, and T. Lange. 2011. Acute sleep deprivation reduces energy expenditure in healthy men. *American Journal of Clinical Nutrition*, 93(6): 1229-1236.

Bickel, W.K., and L.A. Marsch. 2001. Toward a behavioral economic understanding of drug dependence: Delay discounting processes. *Addiction*, 96(1): 73-86.

Bickel, W.K., A.L. Odum, and G.J. Madden. 1999. Impulsivity and cigarette smoking: Delay discounting in current, never, and ex-smokers. *Psychopharmacology*, 146(4): 447-454.

Bilski, J., A. Tełegłów, J. Zahradnik-Bilska, A. Dembin'ski, and Z. Warzecha. 2009. Effects of exercise on appetite and food intake regulation. *Medicina Sportiva*, 13(2): 82-94.

Bosy-Westphal, A., S. Hinrichs, K. Jauch-Chara, B. Hitze, W. Later, B. Wilms, U. Settler, A. Peters, D. Kiosz, and M.J. Müller. 2008. Influence of partial sleep deprivation on energy balance and insulin sensitivity in healthy women. *Obesity Facts*, 1(5): 266-273.

Bryner, R.W., I.H. Ullrich, J. Sauers, J. Donley, G. Hornsby, M. Kolar, and R. Yeater. 1999. Effects of resistance vs. aerobic training combined with an 800 calorie liquid diet on lean body mass and resting metabolic rate. *Journal of the American College of Nutrition*, 18(2): 115-121.

Chardigny, J.M., F. Destaillats, C. Malpuech-Brugère, J. Moulin, D.E. Bauman, A.L. Lock, D.M. Barbano, R.P. Mensink, J.B. Bezelques, P. Chaumont, N. Combe, I. Cristiani, F. Joffre, J.B. German, F. Dionisi, Y. Boirie, and J.L. Sébédio. 2008. Do trans fatty acids from industrially produced sources and from natural sources have the same effect on cardiovascular disease risk factors in healthy subjects? Results of the trans Fatty Acids Collaboration (TRANSFACT) study. *American Journal of Clinical Nutrition*, 87(3): 558-566.

Chtourou, H., and N. Souissi. 2012. The effect of training at a specific time of day: A review. *Journal of Strength and Conditioning Research*, 26(7): 1984-2005.

Cialdini, R.B., R.R. Reno, and C.A. Kallgren. 1990. A focus theory of normative conduct: Recycling the concept of norms to reduce littering in public places. *Journal of Personality and Social Psychology*, 58(6): 1015.

Dankel, S.J., K.T. Mattocks, M.B. Jessee, S.L. Buckner, J.G. Mouser, B.R. Counts, G.C. Laurentino, and J.P. Loenneke. 2016. Frequency: The overlooked resistance training variable for inducing muscle hypertrophy? *Sports Medicine*, October 17 [epub ahead of print].

Dansinger, Michael L., Joi Augustin Gleason, John L. Griffith, Harry P. Selker, and Ernst J. Schaefer. 2005. Comparison of the Atkins, Ornish, Weight Watchers, and Zone diets for weight loss and heart disease risk reduction: A randomized trial. *Jama*, 293(1):43-53.

de Castro, J.M. 2000. Eating behavior: Lessons from the real world of humans. *Nutrition*, 16(10): 800-813.

de Castro, J.M., and E.M. Brewer. 1992. The amount eaten in meals by humans is a power function of the number of people present. *Physiology and Behavior*, 51(1): 121-125.

Dragoni, L. 2005. Understanding the emergence of state goal orientation in organizational work groups: The role of leadership and multilevel climate perceptions. *Journal of Applied Psychology*, 90(6): 1084.

Duhigg, C. 2012. *The power of habit: Why we do what we do in life and business* (vol. 34, no. 10). New York: Random House.

Dweck, C. 2013. *Mindset: The psychology of success.* New York: Random House.

Farshchi, H.R., M.A. Taylor, and I.A. Macdonald. 2004. Decreased thermic effect of food after an irregular compared with a regular meal pattern in healthy lean women. *International Journal of Obesity*, 28(5): 653-660.

Gailliot, M.T., R.F. Baumeister, C.N. DeWall, J.K. Maner, E.A. Plant, D.M. Tice, L.E. Brewer, and B.J. Schmeichel. 2007. Self-control relies on glucose as a limited energy source: Willpower is more than a metaphor. *Journal of Personality and Social Psychology*, 92(2): 325.

Galla, B.M., and A.L. Duckworth. 2015. More than resisting temptation: Beneficial habits mediate the relationship between self-control and positive life outcomes. *Journal of Personality and Social Psychology*, 109(3): 508.

Gibala, M.J., and S.L. McGee. 2008. Metabolic adaptations to short-term high-intensity interval training: A little pain for a lot of gain? *Exercise and Sport Sciences Reviews*, 36(2): 58-63.

Gibson, S.A. 2007. Dietary sugars intake and micronutrient adequacy: A systematic review of the evidence. *Nutrition Research Reviews*, 20(2): 121-131.

Gibson, A.A., R.V. Seimon, C.M.Y. Lee, J. Ayre, J. Franklin, T.P. Markovic, I.D. Caterson, and A. Sainsbury. 2015. Do ketogenic diets really suppress appetite? A systematic review and meta-analysis. *Obesity Reviews*, 16(1): 64-76.

Goldberg, A.L., J.D. Etlinger, D.F. Goldspink, and C. Jablecki. 1974. Mechanism of work-induced hypertrophy of skeletal muscle. *Medicine and Science in Sports*, 7(3): 185-198.

Green, L., A.F. Fry, and J. Myerson. 1994. Discounting of delayed rewards: A life-span comparison. *Psychological Science*, 5(1): 33-36.

Hagger, M.S., and N.L. Chatzisarantis. 2016. Commentary: Misguided effort with elusive implications, and sifting signal from noise with replication science. *Frontiers in Psychology*, 7: 621.

Hall, K.D., T. Bemis, R. Brychta, K.Y. Chen, A. Courville, E.J. Crayner, S. Goodwin, J. Guo, L. Howard, N.D. Knuth, and B.V. Miller. 2015. Calorie for calorie, dietary fat restriction results in more body fat loss than carbohydrate restriction in people with obesity. *Cell Metabolism*, 22(3): 427-436.

Halton, T.L., and F.B. Hu. 2004. The effects of high protein diets on thermogenesis, satiety and weight loss: A critical review. *Journal of the American College of Nutrition*, 23(5): 373-385.

Herman, C.P., D.A. Roth, and J. Polivy. 2003. Effects of the presence of others on food intake: A normative interpretation. *Psychological Bulletin*, 129(6): 873.

Hill, D.W., J.A. Leiferman, N.A. Lynch, B.S. Dangelmaier, and S.E. Burt. 1998. Temporal specificity in adaptations to high-intensity exercise training. *Medicine and Science in Sports and Exercise*, 30(3): 450-455.

Howell, W.H., D.J. McNamara, M.A. Tosca, B.T. Smith, and J.A. Gaines. 1997. Plasma lipid and lipoprotein responses to dietary fat and cholesterol: A meta-analysis. *American Journal of Clinical Nutrition*, 65(6): 1747-1764.

Hsu, M-H., T.L. Ju, C-H. Yen, and C-M. Chang. 2007. Knowledge sharing behavior in virtual communities: The relationship between trust, self-efficacy, and outcome expectations. *International Journal of Human-Computer Studies*, 65(2): 153-169.

Hubal, M.J., H. Gordish-Dressman, P.D. Thompson, T.B. Price, E.P. Hoffman, T.J. Angelopoulos, P.M. Gordon, N.M. Moyna, L.S. Pescatello, P.S. Visich, and R.F. Zoeller. 2005. Variability in muscle size and strength gain after unilateral resistance training. *Medicine and Science in Sports and Exercise*, 37(6): 964-972.

Inzlicht, M., E. Berkman, and N. Elkins-Brown. 2016. The neuroscience of "ego depletion" or: How the brain can help us understand why self-control seems limited. In *Social neuroscience: Biological approaches to social psychology*, ed. E. Harmon-Jones and M. Inzlict, 101-123. New York: Routledge.

Judson, M. n.d. Journalists who were caught lying. *Ranker.* www.ranker.com/list/journalists-who-lied/mel-judson?var=5&utm_expid=16418821-201.EEIZkBszS3O1rZiBcoCRjg.2

Karl, J.P., and S.B. Roberts. 2014. Energy density, energy intake, and body weight regulation in adults. *Advances in Nutrition: An International Review Journal*, 5(6): 835-850.

Killer, S.C., A.K. Blannin, and A.E. Jeukendrup. 2014. No evidence of dehydration with moderate daily coffee intake: A counterbalanced cross-over study in a free-living population. *PloS One*, 9(1): 84154.

Kraemer, W.J., K. Adams, E. Cafarelli, G.A. Dudley, C. Dooly, M.S. Feigenbaum, S.J. Fleck, B. Franklin, A.C. Fry, J.R. Hoffman, R.U. Newton, J. Potteiger, M.H. Stone, N.A. Ratamess, T. Triplett-McBride, and American College of Sports Medicine. 2002. American College of Sports Medicine position stand. Progression models in resistance training for healthy adults. *Medicine and Science in Sports and Exercise*, 34(2): 364-380.

Kraemer, W.J., and N.A. Ratamess. 2005. Hormonal responses and adaptations to resistance exercise and training. *Sports Medicine*, 35(4): 339-361.

Kraft, J.A., J.M. Green, P.A. Bishop, M.T. Richardson, Y.H. Neggers, and J.D. Leeper. 2012. The influence of hydration on anaerobic performance: A review. *Research Quarterly for Exercise and Sport*, 83(2): 282-292.

Kramer, F.M., R.W. Jeffery, J.L. Forster, and M.K. Snell. 1989. Long-term follow-up of behavioral treatment for obesity: Patterns of weight regain among men and women. *International Journal of Obesity*, 13(2): 123-136.

Kuk, J.L., and R. Ross. 2009. Influence of sex on total and regional fat loss in overweight and obese men and women. *International Journal of Obesity*, 33(6): 629-634.

Laforgia, J., R.T. Withers, and C.J. Gore. 2006. Effects of exercise intensity and duration on the excess post-exercise oxygen consumption. *Journal of Sports Sciences*, 24(12): 1247-1264.

Layman, D.K., E. Evans, J.I. Baum, J. Seyler, D.J. Erickson, and R.A. Boileau. 2005. Dietary protein and exercise have additive effects on body composition during weight loss in adult women. *Journal of Nutrition*, 135(8): 1903-1910.

Li, C.S.R., X. Luo, P. Yan, K. Bergquist, and R. Sinha. 2009. Altered impulse control in alcohol dependence: Neural measures of stop signal performance. *Alcoholism: Clinical and Experimental Research*, 33(4): 740-750.

Lichtenstein, A.H., L. Van Horn, and Nutrition Committee. 1998. Very low fat diets. *Circulation*, 98(9): 935-939.

Lissner, L., D.A. Levitsky, B.J. Strupp, H.J. Kalkwarf, and D.A. Roe. 1987. Dietary fat and the regulation of energy intake in human subjects. *American Journal of Clinical Nutrition*, 46(6): 886-892.

Livingstone, M.B.E., J.J. Strain, A.M. Prentice, W.A. Coward, G.B. Nevin, M.E. Barker, R.J. Hickey, P.G. McKenna, and R.G. Whitehead. 1991. Potential contribution of leisure activity to the energy expenditure patterns of sedentary populations. *British Journal of Nutrition*, 65(2): 145-155.

McMillan, D.W., and Chavis, D.M. 1986. Sense of community; A definition and theory. *Journal of Community Psychology*, 14(1): 6-23.

Mohebi-Nejad A. and B. Bikdeli. 2014. Omega-3 supplements and cardiovascular diseases. *Tanaffos,* 13(1): 6.

Monaco, J., A. Mounsey, and J. Bello Kottenstette. 2013. Should you still recommend omega-3 supplements? *The Journal of Family Practice*, 62(8): 422.

Loewenstein, G. 2005. Hot-cold empathy gaps and medical decision making. *Health Psychology* 24(4 Suppl): S49-S56.

Lorente-Cebrián, S., A.G. Costa, S. Navas-Carretero, M. Zabala, J.A. Martínez, and M.J. Moreno-Aliaga. 2013. Role of omega-3 fatty acids in obesity, metabolic syndrome, and cardiovascular diseases: A review of the evidence. *Journal of Physiology and Biochemistry*, 69(3): 633-651.

Marcus, M.D., R.R. Wing, and D.M. Lamparski. 1985. Binge eating and dietary restraint in obese patients. *Addictive Behaviors*, 10(2): 163-168.

Martin, W.F., L.E. Armstrong, and N.R. Rodriguez. 2005. Dietary protein intake and renal function. *Nutrition and Metabolism*, 2(1): 25.

Mattson, M.P., and R. Wan. 2005. Beneficial effects of intermittent fasting and caloric restriction on the cardiovascular and cerebrovascular systems. *Journal of Nutritional Biochemistry*, 16(3): 129-137.

McCann, K.L., M.G. Perri, A.M. Nezu, and M.R. Lowe. 1992. An investigation of counterregulatory eating in obese clinic attenders. *International Journal of Eating Disorders*, 12(2): 161-169.

Milgram, S., L. Bickman, and L. Berkowitz. 1969. Note on the drawing power of crowds of different size. *Journal of Personality and Social Psychology*, 13(2): 79.

Mischel, W., Y. Shoda, and M.I. Rodriguez. 1989. Delay of gratification in children. *Science*, 244(4907): 933-938.

Mozaffarian, D., and R. Clarke. 2009. Quantitative effects on cardiovascular risk factors and coronary heart disease risk of replacing partially hydrogenated vegetable oils with other fats and oils. *European Journal of Clinical Nutrition*, 63: S22-S33.

Naude, C.E., A. Schoonees, M. Senekal, T. Young, P. Garner, and J. Volmink. 2014. Low carbohydrate versus isoenergetic balanced diets for reducing weight and cardiovascular risk: A systematic review and meta-analysis. *PloS One*, 9(7): e100652.

Neal, D.T., W. Wood, J.S. Labrecque, and P. Lally. 2012. How do habits guide behavior? Perceived and actual triggers of habits in daily life. *Journal of Experimental Social Psychology*, 48(2): 492-498.

Nedeltcheva, A.V., J.M. Kilkus, J. Imperial, K. Kasza, D.A. Schoeller, and P.D. Penev. 2009. Sleep curtailment is accompanied by increased intake of calories from snacks. *American Journal of Clinical Nutrition*, 89(1): 126-133.

Norton, L., and G.J. Wilson. 2009. Optimal protein intake to maximize muscle protein synthesis. *AgroFood Industry Hi-Tech*, 20: 54-57.

Ouellette, J.A., and W. Wood. 1998. Habit and intention in everyday life: The multiple processes by which past behavior predicts future behavior. *Psychological Bulletin*, 124(1): 54.

Park, M. 2010. Twinkie diet helps nutrition professor lose 27 pounds. CNN. www.cnn.com/2010/HEALTH/11/08/twinkie.diet.professor/

Perry, C.G., G.J. Heigenhauser, A. Bonen, and L.L. Spriet. 2008. High-intensity aerobic interval training increases fat and carbohydrate metabolic capacities in human skeletal muscle. *Applied Physiology, Nutrition, and Metabolism*, 33(6): 1112-1123.

Pérusse, L., J.P. Despres, S. Lemieux, T. Rice, D.C. Rao, and C. Bouchard. 1996. Familial aggregation of abdominal visceral fat level: Results from the Quebec family study. *Metabolism*, 45(3): 378-382.

Peters, J.C., J. Beck, M. Cardel, H.R. Wyatt, G.D. Foster, Z. Pan, A.C. Wojtanowski, S.S. Vander Veur, S.J. Herring, C. Brill, and J.O. Hill. 2015. The effects of water and non-nutritive sweetened beverages on weight loss and weight maintenance: A randomized clinical trial. *Obesity*, 24(2): 297-304.

Petrella, J.K., J.S. Kim, D.L. Mayhew, J.M. Cross, and M.M. Bamman. 2008. Potent myofiber hypertrophy during resistance training in humans is associated with satellite cell-mediated myonuclear addition: A cluster analysis. *Journal of Applied Physiology*, 104(6): 1736-1742.

Phillips, B. 1999. *Body for life*. New York: HarperCollins.

Phillips, S.M., and L.J. Van Loon. 2011. Dietary protein for athletes: From requirements to optimum adaptation. *Journal of Sports Sciences*, 29(suppl. 1): S29–S38.

Pilcher, J.J., D.R. Ginter, and B. Sadowsky. 1997. Sleep quality versus sleep quantity: Relationships between sleep and measures of health, well-being and sleepiness in college students. *Journal of Psychosomatic Research*, 42(6): 583-596.

Pilcher, J.J., and A.I. Huffcutt. 1996. Effects of sleep deprivation on performance: A meta-analysis. *Sleep*, 19(4): 318-326.

Polivy, J., J. Coleman, and C.P. Herman. 2005. The effect of deprivation on food cravings and eating behavior in restrained and unrestrained eaters. *International Journal of Eating Disorders*, 38(4): 301-309.

Pollock, M.L., and K.R. Vincent. 1996. *Resistance training for health*. President's Council on Physical Fitness and Sports.

Pope, H.G., A.J. Gruber, P. Choi, R. Olivardia, and K.A. Phillips. 1997. Muscle dysmorphia: An underrecognized form of body dysmorphic disorder. *Psychosomatics*, 38(6): 548-557.

Pratley, R., B. Nicklas, M. Rubin, J. Miller, A. Smith, M. Smith, B. Hurley, and A. Goldberg. 1994. Strength training increases resting metabolic rate and norepinephrine levels in healthy 50-to 65-yr-old men. *Journal of Applied Physiology*, 76(1): 133-137.

Ramírez-Campillo, R., D.C. Andrade, C. Campos-Jara, C. Henríquez-Olguín, C. Alvarez-Lepín, and M. Izquierdo. 2013. Regional fat changes induced by localized muscle endurance resistance training. *Journal of Strength and Conditioning Research*, 27(8): 2219-2224.

Reimers, S., E.A. Maylor, N. Stewart, and N. Chater. 2009. Associations between a one-shot delay discounting measure and age, income, education and real-world impulsive behavior. *Personality and Individual Differences*, 47(8): 973-978.

Rolls, B.J., E.T. Rolls, E.A. Rowe, and K. Sweeney. 1981a. Sensory specific satiety in man. *Physiology and Behavior*, 27(1): 137-142.

Rolls, B.J., E.A. Rowe, E.T. Rolls, B. Kingston, A. Megson, and R. Gunary. 1981b. Variety in a meal enhances food intake in man. *Physiology and Behavior*, 26(2): 215-221.

Rosen, I.M., P.A. Gimotty, J.A. Shea, and L.M. Bellini. 2006. Evolution of sleep quantity, sleep deprivation, mood disturbances, empathy, and burnout among interns. *Academic Medicine*, 81(1): 82-85.

Rosen, J.C., and E. Ramirez. 1998. A comparison of eating disorders and body dysmorphic disorder on body image and psychological adjustment. *Journal of Psychosomatic Research*, 44(3): 441-449.

Schachter, S., 1971. Some extraordinary facts about obese humans and rats. *American Psychologist*, 26(2): 129.

Schjerve, I.E., G.A. Tyldum, A.E. Tjønna, T. Stølen, J.P. Loennechen, H.E. Hansen, P.M. Haram, G. Heinrich, A. Bye, S.M. Najjar, and G.L. Smith. 2008. Both aerobic endurance and strength training programmes improve cardiovascular health in obese adults. *Clinical Science*, 115(9): 283-293.

Schoeller, D.A., 2009. The energy balance equation: Looking back and looking forward are two very different views. *Nutrition Reviews*, 67(5): 249-254.

Schoenfeld, B.J. 2010. The mechanisms of muscle hypertrophy and their application to resistance training. *Journal of Strength and Conditioning Research*, 24(10): 2857-2872.

Schoenfeld, B.J., A.A. Aragon, J.W. Krieger, G.T. Sonmez, and C.D. Wilborn. 2014. Body composition changes associated with fasted versus non-fasted aerobic exercise. *Journal of the International Society of Sports Nutrition*, 11(1): 54.

Schoenfeld, B.J., A.A. Aragon, and J.W. Krieger. 2015. Effects of meal frequency on weight loss and body composition: A meta-analysis. *Nutrition Reviews*, 73(2): 69-82.

Schoenfeld, B.J., Z.K. Pope, F.M. Benik, G.M. Hester, J. Sellers, J.L. Nooner, J.A. Schnaiter, K.E. Bond-Williams,

Schoenfeld, B.J., N.A. Ratamess, M.D. Peterson, B. Contreras, and G. Tiryaki-Sonmez. 2015. Influence of resistance training frequency on muscular adaptations in well-trained men. *Journal of Strength and Conditioning Research*, 29(7): 1821-1829.

Selinger, J.C., S.M. O'Connor, J.D. Wong, and J.M. Donelan. 2015. Humans can continuously optimize energetic cost during walking. *Current Biology*, 25(18): 2452-2456.

Sherwood, N.E., R.W. Jeffery, S.A. French, P.J. Hannan, and D.M. Murray. 2000. Predictors of weight gain in the Pound of Prevention study. *International Journal of Obesity*, 24(4): 395-403.

Singh, N.A., K.M. Clements, and M.A. Fiatarone. 1997. A randomized controlled trial of progressive resistance training in depressed elders. *Journals of Gerontology Series A: Biological Sciences and Medical Sciences*, 52(1): M27-M35.

Siri-Tarino, P.W., Q. Sun, F.B. Hu, and R.M. Krauss. 2010. Meta-analysis of prospective cohort studies evaluating the association of saturated fat with cardiovascular disease. *American Journal of Clinical Nutrition*, 91(3): 535-546.

Steele, J. 2014. Intensity; in-ten-si-ty; noun. 1. Often used ambiguously within resistance training. 2. Is it time to drop the term altogether? *British Journal of Sports Medicine*, 48(22): 1586-1588.

Stewart, T.M., D.A. Williamson, and M.A. White. 2002. Rigid vs. flexible dieting: Association with eating disorder symptoms in nonobese women. *Appetite*, 38(1): 39-44.

Taylor, M.A., and J.S. Garrow. 2001. Compared with nibbling, neither gorging nor a morning fast affect short-term energy balance in obese patients in a chamber calorimeter. *International Journal of Obesity and Related Metabolic Disorders*, 25(4): 519

Thomas, M., H. Sing, G. Belenky, H. Holcomb, H. Mayberg, R. Dannals, J.R. Wagner, D. Thorne, K. Popp, L. Rowland, and A. Welsh. 2000. Neural basis of alertness and cognitive performance impairments during sleepiness. I. Effects of 24 h of sleep deprivation on waking human regional brain activity. *Journal of Sleep Research*, 9(4): 335-352.

Thorndike, A.N., L. Sonnenberg, J. Riis, S. Barraclough, and D.E. Levy. 2012. A 2-phase labeling and choice architecture intervention to improve healthy food and beverage choices. *American Journal of Public Health*, 102(3): 527-533.

Trapp, E.G., D.J. Chisholm, J. Freund, and S.H. Boutcher. 2008. The effects of high-intensity intermittent exercise training on fat loss and fasting insulin levels of young women. *International Journal of Obesity*, 32(4): 684-691.

Tremblay, A., J.A. Simoneau, and C. Bouchard. 1994. Impact of exercise intensity on body fatness and skeletal muscle metabolism. *Metabolism*, 43(7): 814-818.

van Strien, T., C.P. Herman, and M.W. Verheijden. 2014. Dietary restraint and body mass change. A 3-year follow up study in a representative Dutch sample. *Appetite*, 76: 44-49.

USDA and UDHHS. 2010. *Report of the Dietary Guidelines Advisory Committee on the dietary guidelines for Americans, 2010*. June 15, 2010. www.cnpp.usda.gov/DGAs2010-DGACReport.htm

Venkatesan, M. 1966. Experimental study of consumer behavior conformity and independence. *Journal of Marketing Research*, 3(4): 384-387.

Vispute, S.S., J.D. Smith, J.D. LeCheminant, and K.S. Hurley. 2011. The effect of abdominal exercise on abdominal fat. *Journal of Strength and Conditioning Research*, 25(9): 2559-2564.

Wakahara, T., A. Fukutani, Y. Kawakami, and T. Yanai. 2013. Non-uniform muscle hypertrophy: Its relation to muscle activation in training session. *Medicine and Science in Sports and Exercise*, 45(11): 2158-2165.

Wansink, B. 2004. Environmental factors that increase the food intake and consumption volume of unknowing consumers. *Annual Review of Nutrition*, 24: 455-479.

Wansink, B., and J. Painter. 2005. Proximity's influence on estimated and actual candy consumption. *Obesity Research*, 13: A204.

Wansink, B., J.E. Painter, and Y.K. Lee. 2006. The office candy dish: Proximity's influence on estimated and actual consumption. *International Journal of Obesity*, 30(5): 871-875.

Wansink, B., and C.R. Payne. 2007. Counting bones: Environmental cues that decreased food intake. *Perceptual and Motor Skills*, 104(1): 273-276.

Wansink, B., and C.R. Payne. 2008. Eating behavior and obesity at Chinese buffets. *Obesity*, 16(8): 1957-1960.

Wansink, B., and J. Sobal. 2007. Mindless eating the 200 daily food decisions we overlook. *Environment and Behavior*, 39(1): 106-123.

Weingarten, H.P. 1984. Meal initiation controlled by learned cues: Basic behavioral properties. *Appetite*, 5(2): 147-158.

Weller, R.E., E.W. Cook, K.B. Avsar, and J.E. Cox. 2008. Obese women show greater delay discounting than healthy-weight women. *Appetite*, 51(3): 563-569.

Wemple, E. 2015. The Brian Williams scandal is an NBC News-wide scandal. *Washington Post*. www.washingtonpost.com/blogs/erik-wemple/wp/2015/02/05/the-brian-williams-scandal-is-an-nbc-news-wide-scandal

Westcott, W.L. 2012. Resistance training is medicine: Effects of strength training on health. *Current Sports Medicine Reports*, 11(4): 209-216.

Westman, Eric C., William S. Yancy, Joel S. Edman, Keith F. Tomlin, and Christine E. Perkins. 2002. Effect of 6-month adherence to a very low carbohydrate diet program. *The American Journal of Medicine*, 113(1): 30-36.

Winett, R.A., and R.N. Carpinelli. 2001. Potential health-related benefits of resistance training. *Preventive Medicine*, 33(5): 503-513.

Wood, W., and D.T. Neal. 2007. A new look at habits and the habit-goal interface. *Psychological Review*, 114(4): 843.

Wood, W., J.M. Quinn, and D.A. Kashy. 2002. Habits in everyday life: Thought, emotion, and action. *Journal of Personality and Social Psychology*, 83(6): 1281.

Yamaguchi, T., and K. Ishii. 2005. Effects of static stretching for 30 seconds and dynamic stretching on leg extension power. *Journal of Strength and Conditioning Research*, 19(3): 677-683.

INDEX

ABOUT THE AUTHOR

Sohee Lee, CSCS, CISSN, is a health coach, researcher, and author who specializes in helping women develop healthy relationships with food and their bodies while reaching their fitness goals. She is pursuing her master's degree in psychology at Arizona State University and earned her bachelor's degree in human biology from Stanford University. Lee is interested in how the field of behavioral psychology can benefit the health and fitness industry.

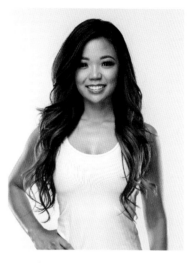

Lee is certified as a strength and conditioning specialist through the National Strength and Conditioning Association (NSCA-CSCS), as a sports nutritionist through the International Society of Sports Nutrition (CISSN), and as a Strong First Girya (SFG) Level I instructor. She has trained clients at elite gyms such as Peak Performance (New York, New York), Cressey Sports Performance (Hudson, Massachusetts), and Tyler English Fitness (Avon, Connecticut) and has established her own fitness center, SoheeFit Systems (Phoenix, Arizona).

Having battled anorexia and bulimia, Lee knows firsthand the toll disordered eating can take on a life. She seeks to explore the psychology behind habits and behavior change, particularly as they relate to food and exercise. Her mission is to empower women to practice compassion and grace with themselves in the gym, in the kitchen, and in life. A professional bikini competitor through the International Fitness Professionals Association (IFPA) federation and an amateur powerlifter, Lee lends her inspirational perspective to major fitness outlets including *Oxygen Magazine*, LIVESTRONG.com, and Bodybuilding.com. She self-published *The Beginner's Guide to Macros* and *Reverse Dieting* and is coauthor of *The Beginner's Guide to Bikini Competitions*. She also cohosts *Physique Science Radio* with Dr. Layne Norton and maintains an active presence on social media. To find out more about Sohee, visit her website, www.soheefit.com.

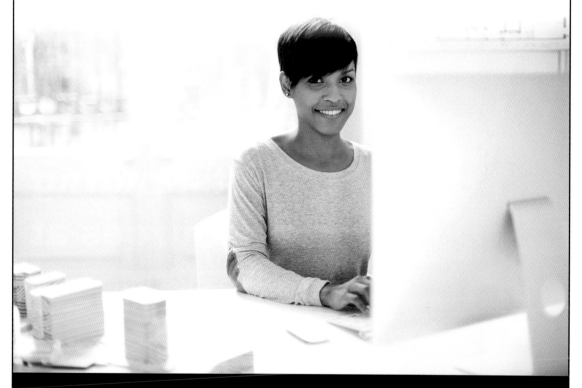
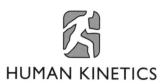

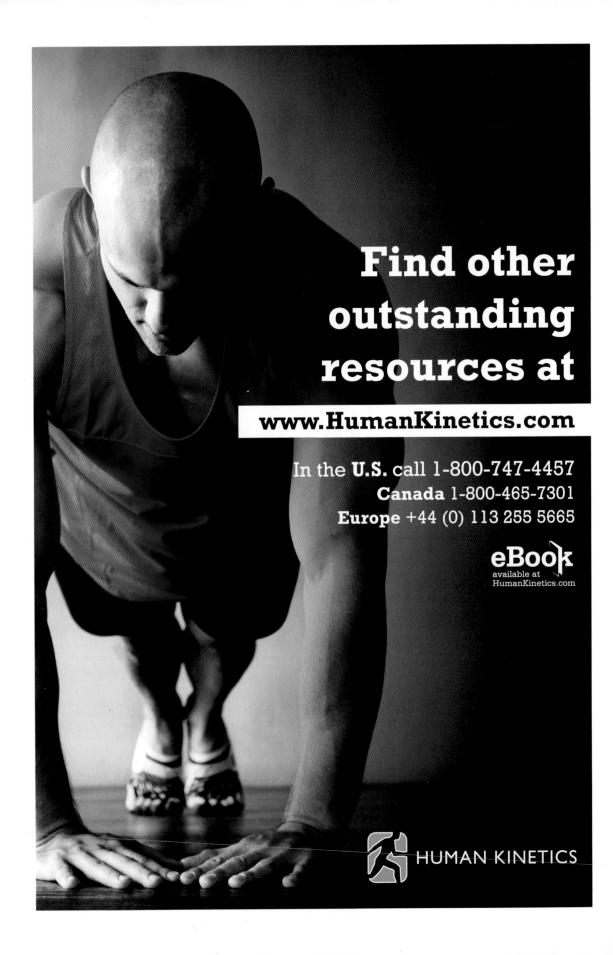